Techniques in Minimally Invasive Thoracic Surgery

Kwhanmien Kim • Seokjin Haam
Hyun Koo Kim
Editors

Techniques in Minimally Invasive Thoracic Surgery

Springer

Editors
Kwhanmien Kim
Department of Thoracic and Cardiovascular Surgery
Seoul National University Bundang Hospital
Seongnam, Republic of Korea

Seokjin Haam
Department of Thoracic and Cardiovascular Surgery
Ajou University Hospital
Suwon, Republic of Korea

Hyun Koo Kim
Department of Thoracic and Cardiovascular Surgery
Korea University Guro Hospital
Seoul, Republic of Korea

ISBN 978-981-19-2474-3 ISBN 978-981-19-2472-9 (eBook)
https://doi.org/10.1007/978-981-19-2472-9

This Springer imprint is published by the registered company Springer Nature Singapore Pte Ltd.
The registered company address is: 152 Beach Road, #21-01/04 Gateway East, Singapore 189721, Singapore

Preface

In Korea, video-assisted thoracic surgery (VATS) was first used to treat pneumothorax in 1992. Thereafter, VATS lobectomy was introduced in Korea in a patient with benign lung disease in 1993. The first anatomical VATS lobectomy with complete mediastinal lymph node dissection was performed on a lung cancer patient in 2003 by Kwhanmien Kim, one of the editors of this book. Since then, VATS has rapidly replaced open thoracotomies and has become the dominant procedure in Korea through the well-designed training program formulated by the Korean Association of Thoracic Surgical Oncology (KATSO). Furthermore, robot-assisted thoracic surgery (RATS) has emerged as an alternative procedure for treating esophageal cancer, mediastinal tumor, and lung cancer. The surgical techniques developed by Korean thoracic surgeons have spread globally and received recognition owing to the enthusiasm of some pioneers and well-established training programs.

Techniques in Minimally Invasive Thoracic Surgery is not intended to be a textbook of thoracic surgery. Instead, this book is designed to provide readers with a wide range of sound techniques and efficient measures that have proved safe and effective in our experience. *Techniques in Minimally Invasive Thoracic Surgery* comprises the three most popular thoracic surgery sections: pulmonary resections, esophagectomy and thymectomy by VATS or RATS and the management of postoperative complications, and nonintubated thoracic surgery. The editors and contributors have ably met their goal of informing the reader about accurate surgical principles needed to treat thoracic diseases.

We would like to gratefully acknowledge the favor of authors who are members of KATSO. Without their dedication and sponsorship from KATSO, this book could not have been compiled. We hope that *Techniques in Minimally Invasive Thoracic Surgery* will help readers consolidate their understanding of surgical procedures and promote their technical standards to a higher level.

Seongnam, Republic of Korea — Kwhanmien Kim
Suwon, Republic of Korea — Seokjin Haam
Seoul, Republic of Korea — Hyun Koo Kim

Contents

Part II Esophagus

Part III Others

Part I

Lung

Establishment of a Minimally Invasive Thoracic Surgery Program

1

Jong Ho Cho

Abstract

The establishment of minimally invasive surgery is a complex and difficult task. Video-assisted thoracic surgery (VATS) refers to a minimally invasive surgical technique that represents a less invasive approach to thoracic surgery using thoracoscopy. For lung cancer or esophageal cancer surgery, planning and establishing a team for minimally invasive surgery for the first time is not a simple task. Technical advances in surgical devices and the enhanced skill of surgeons are cornerstones of the development of minimally invasive surgery. Here, we review the meaning of minimally invasive thoracic surgery and discuss how to establish a team approach for VATS procedures.

Keywords

Video-assisted thoracic surgery · Minimally invasive surgery · Surgery

J. H. Cho (✉)
Department of Thoracic and Cardiovascular Surgery, Samsung Medical Center, Sungkyunkwan University School of Medicine, Seoul, Republic of Korea
e-mail: jongho9595.cho@samsung.com

1.1 Introduction

In recent years, there has been a shift towards video-assisted thoracic surgery (VATS) in the field of thoracic surgery. VATS refers to surgery to remove lung cancer, esophageal cancer, or mediastinal tumors without rib cutting or sternotomy, as was done in the past. In general, minimally invasive surgery is associated with less pain, shorter hospital stays, and fewer complications [1]. It also has allowed surgeons to perform new, complex, and conventional procedures without the major risks associated with a large open incision.

VATS is just one of the first types of minimally invasive surgery. One subtype of minimally invasive surgery is robotic surgery, which offers surgeons a magnified, three-dimensional view of the surgical site with better flexibility and control. We can use these advanced robotic surgical techniques to achieve excellent surgical outcomes and safety in most cases of thoracic surgery.

The technical and oncological safety of thoracoscopic surgery for early-stage lung cancer is considered acceptable worldwide [2, 3]. It has recently been reported that the majority of thoracic surgical procedures can be performed with minimal invasive surgery due to advances in the development of surgical techniques, even in complex cases of patients with lung cancer [4]. However, even with minimally invasive surgery,

K. Kim et al. (eds.), *Techniques in Minimally Invasive Thoracic Surgery*,
https://doi.org/10.1007/978-981-19-2472-9_1

there are risks of complications involving anesthesia, major bleeding, and infection [5]. Therefore, it is important to prepare for serious complications, such as massive bleeding from the pulmonary artery during VATS, with a backup plan always in mind [6].

1.2 How to Set Up an Excellent Surgical Team for Minimally Invasive Surgery

Team Approach

It is unusual for patients to receive more attention from the medical team than during surgery. Patients are prepared by 1 surgeon, 1 or 2 assistants, anesthesiologists, and nursing staff. Each member of the surgical team has his or her own function, but the surgical team is like playing a symphony, so each team member must collaborate with his or her colleagues to achieve good results. The patient's life is in the hands of the operating team, so there can be no such thing as properness for its own sake in the operating room. To bring the best results for the patient, everyone must work quickly and effectively, often in desperate situations. They need to be familiar with surgical procedures, how to operate machines (e.g., surgical robot systems), instruments, and surgical items, understand each other, trust each other, cooperate, and be considerate. A person who does not devote his or her whole heart to working as a good member of the team, and who instead tries to work at his own level, creates dissonance in teamwork, making it difficult to work together in the operating room.

A surgical team includes an array of specialists who need to work in close cooperation for the operation to succeed. A single error, miscommunication, or slow response can have disastrous consequences. To develop the best surgical team, we have to be the best possible leader. An excellent article on the approach to building a surgical team approach was published in the *Harvard Business Review* [7]. They presented several factors for the development of a successful team, as described below.

Creating a Learning Team

The surgeon as a team leader should follow the up-to-date knowledge in secondary medical textbooks, quickly acquire new medical skills, share them with fellow doctors, and build a system while maintaining the 4 components of team works [7]. The new paradigm of health care focuses increasingly on interdisciplinary teams as its core unit. The increasing complexity of the surgical environment has changed the delivery of surgical care and has increasingly led to the formation of multidisciplinary provider teams replacing the more traditional individualistic surgeon–assistant–nurse relationship. The challenges are considerable, even if we are already faced with tight competition, especially in the 80-h working-week environment of surgical resident programs. It may be a good strategy for surgical educators to collaborate with other colleagues who have conducted training for a certain period.

Framing the Challenge

Properly framing the challenge is critical to our success in the field of surgery. A frame challenge is where someone answers a question in a wholly different way that the asker never expected, but in a way that he or she feels will solve the problem. The difficulty of introducing new surgical procedures places more stress on team members than usual for minimally invasive surgery. Surgeons must help their team embrace and internalize the legitimacy of this important new challenge regarding new surgical techniques. Even so, identifying the right challenge for innovation is particularly crucial for the surgical team.

Creating an Environment of Psychological Safety That Fosters Communication and Innovation

It is important to have an environment where the leader's innovation and creativity are properly accepted, and team members can exchange feedback with each other. A belief that one will not be punished or humiliated for speaking up with ideas, questions, or mistakes is important for both a leader and team members. This relates to assistants feeling empowered to express an idea or contribution fully, without fear of negative consequences to themselves or their status [7]. It includes being courageous enough to own one's mistakes and turn them into learning, and to trust that one's work environment and co-workers will not shame one for doing so [7].

Preparation

It is important to always prepare the basic rules of surgery, the instruments used, the order of surgery, and the materials for surgery. To pack all the items to be prepared before surgery, possible surgical materials and instruments should be listed and prepared.

Surgical practice has evolved rapidly, driven in part by the increasing complexity of patients, the severity of their diseases, rapidly evolving new technologies, and a deluge of evidence to support best practices. For example, the application of robotic surgical systems for lobectomy was first described in 2002 [8]. Since then, robotic-assisted VATS lobectomy has become more popular for the treatment of lung cancer, and the rapid evolution of technology has prompted many centers to initiate robotic surgical procedures [9, 10].

Prepare for the Worst, Hope for the Best

> Great deeds are usually wrought at great risks
> —Herodotus (484–402 B.C.)

Conversion to Thoracotomy or Sternotomy

If one has to switch to thoracotomy or sternotomy from VATS, one should not hesitate. Surgeons must always be ready for the possibility of open conversion and should rehearse this possibility with team members. For VATS lobectomy, the incidence of intraoperative conversion to an open approach ranges from 5 to 23%, and nearly half the conversions are performed emergently [11, 12]. In fact, the surgeon should set his or her appropriate criteria for conversion to open thoracotomy or sternotomy. For example, Dunning and Walker [13] suggested that a surgical team should use a reasonable parameter for the timing of conversion, which may be if the pulmonary artery has not been divided within 1.5–2 h.

Management of Intraoperative Bleeding

Although an increasing number of studies have found that VATS lobectomy appears to be superior to conventional open lobectomy for perioperative outcomes [1, 14], even minimally invasive surgery still involves risks for intraoperative complications such as intraoperative bleeding. A major concern in VATS procedures is that trying to dissect a pulmonary vessel or another large vessel during the surgery may lead to severe bleeding, which is troublesome to control with small ports. Surgeons should keep a sponge stick available to immediately apply pressure to control bleeding when it happens. Here are the author's own safety rules to manage massive bleeding during VATS lobectomy:

Management when massive bleeding occurs during VATS lobectomy

1. Ask for help: anesthesiologist, cardiac surgeon, or senior thoracic surgeon.
2. Blood transfusion: ask for a massive transfusion from nursing staff or others.
3. Calm down and compress: control your own heartbeat, prepare a sponge stick, and immediately apply pressure with it.
4. Decide whether thoracotomy is really needed.
5. Expose the main pulmonary trunk or proximal part of the injured vessel.
6. Fix the injured vessel with a suture or fibrin sealant patch.

Check Possible Clues to Prevent Reoperation Before Leaving the Operating Room After Surgery

Before leaving the operating room, it is necessary to make sure that the entire surgical procedure has been performed well. Especially before closing after lung cancer surgery, it is necessary to check several factors to prevent postoperative complications such as bronchopleural fistula, torsion, bleeding, and prolonged air leak. Below is a list of the items that the author always must verify before leaving the operating room after lobectomy.

Checklist before leaving the operating room after lobectomy

1. Airway: check the bronchial stump.
2. Bleeding: check the vascular stump (pulmonary artery/vein, bronchial artery) and incision site.
3. Circulation: check venous drainage.
4. Drain: check the appropriate position of the chest tube or catheter.
5. Expansion: check that there is enough pulmonary expansion.
6. Fissure: check for a complete fissure (possible torsion).

Record the Quality Notes and Feedback

Furthermore, surgeons must keep meticulous perioperative notes and record a quality report, which is mandatory for all new surgical procedures. Defining and measuring how each of a variety of factors affects outcomes is an important but challenging objective. As for perioperative complications, the procedure and process during which they occurred, how the results appeared, and the resulting solutions should be recorded in detail so that the procedure can develop as experience is accumulated. Based on these records, more complex surgical procedures can be performed using minimally invasive surgery, as is happening in the field at this moment.

1.3 Conclusion

Surgeons should constantly think about why we do minimally invasive surgery and look at it from the patient's point of view. Of course, it is acceptable for any surgeon to pursue minimally invasive surgery because it can provide the patient with better surgical outcomes, such as a quicker recovery and fewer complications. However, surgeons may try to avoid minimally invasive surgery in complicated and difficult cases. Minimally invasive surgery requires some risk and preparation to be successful. We must constantly work with our team members to continue developing our surgical skills, easily adapt to new equipment, and use new techniques freely.

Lastly, I would like to share with you the saying by Professor Young Mog Shim, my teacher and mentor:

> Surgery should be done using the best surgical method for the patient, not a comfortable and easy surgery for the surgeon.

Conflict of Interest No potential conflict of interest relevant to this article was reported.

References

1. Nwogu CE, D'Cunha J, Pang H, et al. VATS lobectomy has better perioperative outcomes than open lobectomy: CALGB 31001, an ancillary analysis of CALGB 140202 (Alliance). Ann Thorac Surg. 2015;99:399–405.
2. Swanson SJ, Herndon JE 2nd, D'Amico TA, et al. Video-assisted thoracic surgery lobectomy: report of CALGB 39802: a prospective, multi-institution feasibility study. J Clin Oncol. 2007;25:4993–7.
3. Yan TD, Black D, Bannon PG, McCaughan BC. Systematic review and meta-analysis of randomized and nonrandomized trials on safety and efficacy of video-assisted thoracic surgery lobectomy for early-stage non-small-cell lung cancer. J Clin Oncol. 2009;27:2553–62.
4. Solli P, Bertolaccini L, Droghetti A, et al. 2016 Annual report from the Italian VATS Group. Future Oncol. 2018;14(6s):23–8.
5. Boffa DJ, Kosinski AS, Furnary AP, et al. Minimally invasive lung cancer surgery performed by thoracic surgeons as effective as thoracotomy. J Clin Oncol. 2018;36:2378–85.
6. Liang C, Wen H, Guo Y, et al. Severe intraoperative complications during VATS lobectomy compared with thoracotomy lobectomy for early stage non-small cell lung cancer. J Thorac Dis. 2013;5:513–7.
7. Edmondson A, Bohmer R, Pisano G. Speeding up team learning. Harv Bus Rev. 2001;79:125–32.
8. Melfi FM, Menconi GF, Mariani AM, Angeletti CA. Early experience with robotic technology for thoracoscopic surgery. Eur J Cardiothorac Surg. 2002;21:864–8.

9. Moller T, Egberts JH, Eichhorn M, et al. Current status and evolution of robotic-assisted thoracic surgery in Germany-results from a nationwide survey. J Thorac Dis. 2019;11:4807–15.
10. Zirafa CC, Romano G, Key TH, Davini F, Melfi F. The evolution of robotic thoracic surgery. Ann Cardiothorac Surg. 2019;8:210–7.
11. Lim CG, Shin KM, Lim JS, et al. Predictors of conversion to thoracotomy during video-assisted thoracoscopic surgery lobectomy in lung cancer: additional predictive value of FDG-PET/CT in a tuberculosis endemic region. J Thorac Dis. 2017;9:2427–36.
12. Samson P, Guitron J, Reed MF, Hanseman DJ, Starnes SL. Predictors of conversion to thoracotomy for video-assisted thoracoscopic lobectomy: a retrospective analysis and the influence of computed tomography-based calcification assessment. J Thorac Cardiovasc Surg. 2013;145:1512–8.
13. Dunning J, Walker WS. How to set up a VATS lobectomy program. Ann Cardiothorac Surg. 2012;1:43–6.
14. Puri V, Patel A, Majumder K, et al. Intraoperative conversion from video-assisted thoracoscopic surgery lobectomy to open thoracotomy: a study of causes and implications. J Thorac Cardiovasc Surg. 2015;149:55–62.

Video-Assisted Thoracic Surgery Wedge Resection for Primary Spontaneous Pneumothorax

2

Duk Hwan Moon, Bong Jun Kim, Wongi Woo, and Sungsoo Lee

Abstract

Primary spontaneous pneumothorax (PSP) is most commonly treated using VATS wedge resection or bullectomy in many institutions. Herein, a broad overview of VATS, along with its various techniques, including their respective benefits and disadvantages, in treating PSP is provided with some recommendations. Additionally, resected site coverage techniques and materials are also discussed, as there is increasing evidence suggesting that this may have greater impact on recurrence rate than surgical techniques.

2.1 Introduction

Among patients who had primary spontaneous pneumothorax (PSP), recurrence is very common. In many institutions, surgical treatment, such as bullectomy or wedge resection, is most often considered for the management of PSP recurrence [1, 2]. In some cases, however, nonsurgical treatment such as endo-loop ligation or pleurodesis can also be considered [3, 4]. Nonetheless, surgical approach is considered to be the most effective treatment in minimizing the risk of another recurrence in patients with prior PSP. In the realm of surgical treatments, there is substantial evidence suggesting that minimally invasive approach, such as video-assisted thoracic surgery (VATS), is preferred to the conventional, non-minimally invasive techniques, such as thoracotomy. This is because the former has been shown to reduce postoperative pain and recovery time, allowing speedy return to normal physical activities. Moreover, VATS has also shown to provide better respiratory function when compared with thoracotomy. Since Schramel et al. published a paper on VATS pneumothorax surgery in 1996, almost all surgical treatments of PSP were done using VATS; and in fact, it would be safe to assert that all thoracic surgeons would unanimously choose VATS to treat PSP [5]. Due to recent developments in surgical instruments and anesthetic techniques, VATS—for the purpose of treating PSP—can be carried out either via single-port or multiport incisions and either by awakening or non-intubated techniques.

2.2 PSP Surgical Indication

Although recurrent PSP is generally an indication of surgical treatment, many institutions nonetheless have begun using VATS even for first-event PSP because it has become so widely

D. H. Moon · B. J. Kim · W. Woo · S. Lee (✉)
Department of Thoracic and Cardiovascular Surgery, Gangnam Severance Hospital, Yonsei University College of Medicine, Seoul, Republic of Korea
e-mail: CHESTLEE@yuhs.ac

K. Kim et al. (eds.), *Techniques in Minimally Invasive Thoracic Surgery*,
https://doi.org/10.1007/978-981-19-2472-9_2

accepted and universalized. Moreover, because it has been reported that the recurrence rate of PSP is greater than 70%, if bullae are identified clearly on chest computed tomography (CT) or chest X-ray, then VATS bullectomy or VATS wedge resection is performed to easily and simply reduce the recurrence rate [2]. Additionally, the following can be considered as indications for surgical treatment: bilateral PSP, persistent air leak for 4–5 days, accompanied by conditions that could cause hemodynamic compromise, such as tension pneumothorax or hemothorax, and cases of failure to completely re-expand the lung, as well as risks that could impact the lifestyle and profession. However, to the best of our knowledge, there is no prospective randomized study regarding this point. Such a study on a large scale may be difficult due to the nature of the disease and ethical concerns.

2.3 PSP Surgery Using VATS

The intercostal space is opened up by positioning the patients in lateral decubitus posture, with or without having the operating table flexed at 30° (Fig. 2.1). Currently, the most common technique of VATS is performed using three ports; one placed at the seventh intercostal space mid-axillary line, one placed at the fourth intercostal space anterior axillary line, and another placed just anterior to the tip of the scapula. This triangular setup allows for a full panoramic view of the pleural cavity, and if the ports are spaced apart adequately, it prevents instrument collision (Fig. 2.2). Of course, placement of the port site is dependent on the preference of the surgeon, and the port size is dependent on the size of the camera and instruments.

The entire pleural cavity must be inspected first using atraumatic blunt instruments (forceps) to manipulate the lung tissues. All adhesions should be removed using endoscopic instruments to ensure good operating field. Although most ruptured bullae are located on the apex of the

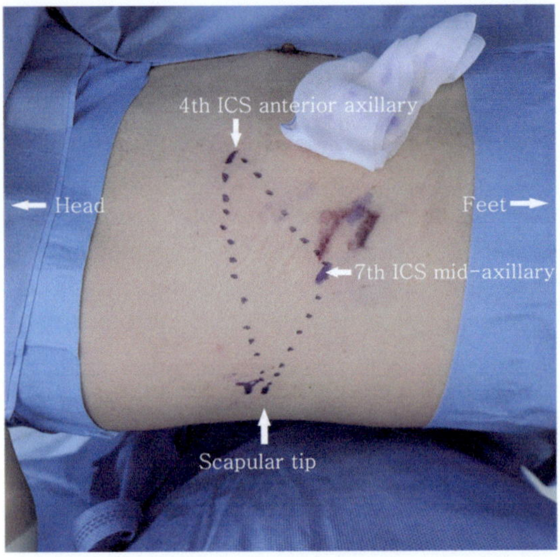

Fig. 2.2 Ports location for the three ports technique. *ICS* intercostal space

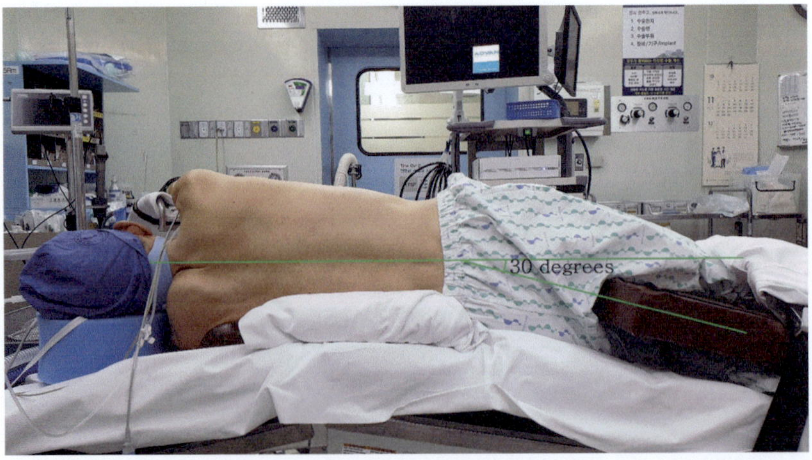

Fig. 2.1 During VATS surgery, the operating table is flexed at 30° to widen the intercostal space and facilitate the operation of the thoracoscopic instruments

upper lobe or on the superior segment of the lower lobe, thorough inspection of the entire lung surface is recommended.

Endoscopic bullectomy is performed using endo-staplers. To prevent air leakage, the resection line should be across the healthy lung tissues and the staples should not cross one another. Additionally, when performing wedge resection, the shape of the lung is an important consideration. The lung, when ventilated, must unfold and expand smoothly in a shape similar to that of before surgery. In other words, if resection is done with an inappropriate shape, then the lung, when ventilated, will expand awkwardly and improperly, potentially causing postoperative pleural adhesion, which contribute to recurrence and diminished lung function. In the case of subpleural bleb, ball-tip abrasion may be used (Fig. 2.3); and in the case of small single bulla, endo-loop technique is used for ligation. It is important to proceed gently with caution during bullectomy to avert damages and tearing to the lung. Chest tubes—one or two, depending on the circumstances—are inserted through the ports after confirming successful hemostasis and observing no air leakage from the staple line. Chest tubes insertion should be done in the direction toward the apex and placed antero-laterally in the pleural cavity. The lung is then reinflated under direct vision and the wounds are closed. Depending on the surgeon's preference, small bore tubes or flexible drain catheters may be used instead of the classic chest tube.

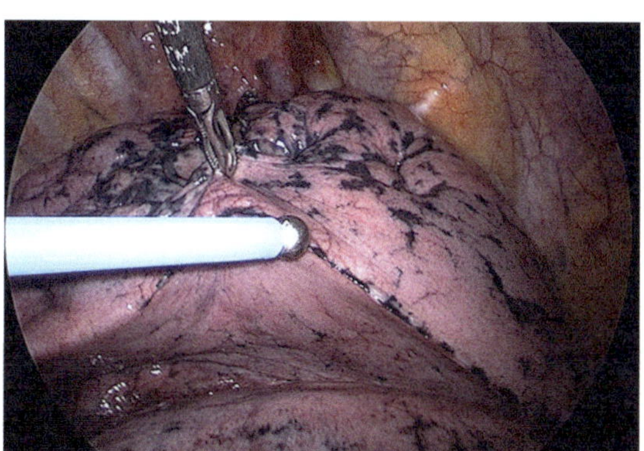

Fig. 2.3 In the case of a subpleural bleb, abrasion using a ball-tip can be performed

Since Rocco and colleagues announced positive results of single-port VATS for treating pneumothorax in 2004, this technique has been adopted by many institutions [6]. Single-port VATS is considered to be safe, with many added benefits, including reduced postoperative pain. However, despite the benefits of single-port VATS compared with the conventional three-port VATS, the single-port technique requires a steep learning curve, and in fact, may be disadvantageous in that due to comparatively lower access points, a full scan may not be as easy and possible during lung and diaphragm inspection. However, with the advancements made recently to surgical instruments, and with adequate surgical experience, the single-port technique may be a promising alternative to the traditional three-port VATS, with great hopes and expectations from the thoracic surgery community.

2.4 PSP Recurrence After VATS

With the introduction of VATS, great strides have been made in pneumothorax surgery. Compared with the traditional open thoracotomy, minimally invasive approach has shown improvements in postoperative bleeding, degree of postoperative pain, chest tube indwelling time, and duration of hospital stay. However, recurrence still remains to be improved, and thus, a challenge to be addressed [7–9].

To date, there have been many studies evaluating the various surgical treatment methods for managing postoperative recurrence; such techniques include pleurodesis, pleural abrasion, pleurectomy, etc. However, recent studies suggest that the coverage technique and materials applied to the stapling sites may also influence the risk of recurrence [10]. There is increased evidence suggesting that using an oxidized regenerated cellulose (ORC) sheet or polyglycolic acid (PGA) sheet to cover the resected site may provide benefits. Based on a recent systematic review, appropriate coverage materials and technique may provide greater benefit than the various benefits from surgical techniques, like mechanical and chemical pleurodesis [10]. In addition, a recent meta-analysis evaluating the coverage material showed that PGA sheet coverage may reduce the recurrence rate [11]. Moreover, the benefits of vicryl mesh was also shown in a recent randomized controlled trial [12]. However, at the moment, there is no clear consensus and definition, at least temporally during the postoperative period, of what constitutes a recurrence. Some assert that within a window of 30 days after surgery is part of the healing process of the stapling site [13]. Also, it is believed that postoperative recurrence of pneumothorax may be attributable to neo-bullae genesis [13, 14]. In line with this, many thoracic surgeons are in consensus that covering this area with coverage material may be important.

2.5 Conclusions

Minimally invasive surgery, like VATS, is a popular surgical treatment for PSP. With further advancements in surgical instruments and endostaplers, single-port VATS may be a promising alternative to the traditional multiport technique. Nonetheless, to minimize the risk of postoperative recurrence, careful inspection of the full lung surface is highly recommended, and of course, it is important to diligently build surgical experience.

References

1. Nonomura R, Tabata T. Re-operation for recurrent spontaneous pneumothorax. Kyobu geka Jpn J Thorac Surg. 2021;74(10):833–8.
2. Porcel JM, Lee P. Thoracoscopy for spontaneous pneumothorax. J Clin Med. 2021;10(17):3835.
3. Lee YM, Lim YC, Liam CK, Aljafri M. Video-assisted thoracoscopic surgery for pneumothorax. Med J Malays. 1995;50(4):334–8.
4. Liu YH, Chao YK, Wu YC, et al. Bullae ablation in primary spontaneous pneumothorax. World J Surg. 2009;33(5):938–42.
5. Schramel FM, Sutedja TG, Braber JC, van Mourik JC, Postmus PE. Cost-effectiveness of video-assisted thoracoscopic surgery versus conservative treatment for first time or recurrent spontaneous pneumothorax. Eur Respir J. 1996;9(9):1821–5.
6. Rocco G, Martin-Ucar A, Passera E. Uniportal VATS wedge pulmonary resections. Ann Thorac Surg. 2004;77(2):726–8.
7. Cardillo G, Bintcliffe OJ, Carleo F, et al. Primary spontaneous pneumothorax: a cohort study of VATS with talc poudrage. Thorax. 2016;71(9):847–53.
8. Hirai K, Kawashima T, Takeuchi S, Usuda J. Covering the staple line with a polyglycolic acid sheet after bullectomy for primary spontaneous pneumothorax prevents postoperative recurrent pneumothorax. J Thorac Dis. 2015;7(11):1978–85.
9. Hong KP, Kim DK, Kang KH. Staple line coverage with a polyglycolic acid patch and fibrin glue without pleural abrasion after thoracoscopic bullectomy for primary spontaneous pneumothorax. Korean J Thorac Cardiovasc Surg. 2016;49(2):85–91.
10. Asban A, Raza SS, McLeod C, Donahue J, Wei B. Mechanical or chemical and mechanical pleurodesis for spontaneous pneumothorax: what is the most effective approach in preventing recurrence? A systematic review and meta-analysis. Eur J Cardiothorac Surg. 2020;58(4):682–91.
11. Kadomatsu Y, Fukui T, Mori S, Chen-Yoshikawa TF, Wakai K. Polyglycolic acid sheet covering to prevent recurrence after surgery for spontaneous pneumothorax: a meta-analysis. Sci Rep. 2021;11(1):3392.
12. Hsu HH, Liu YH, Chen HY, et al. Vicryl mesh coverage reduced recurrence after bullectomy for primary spontaneous pneumothorax. Ann Thorac Surg. 2021;112(5):1609–15.
13. Onuki T, Kawamura T, Kawabata S, Yamaoka M, Inagaki M. Neo-generation of neogenetic bullae after surgery for spontaneous pneumothorax in young adults: a prospective study. J Cardiothorac Surg. 2019;14(1):20.
14. Ota H, Kawai H, Kuriyama S. The presence of a reticulated trabecula-like structure increases the risk for the recurrence of primary spontaneous pneumothorax after thoracoscopic bullectomy. Ann Thorac Cardiovasc Surg. 2016;22(3):139–45.

3 Surgical Planning and the Division of the Intersegmental Plane During Thoracoscopic Segmentectomy

Ha Eun Kim, Young Ho Yang, and Chang Young Lee

Abstract

Although lobectomy remains the gold-standard surgical treatment for non-small-cell lung cancer, the frequency of thoracoscopic segmentectomy is increasing. Multiple factors must be considered in the choice of the procedure, ranging from adequate surgical planning or simulation, tumor localization, and identification of the intersegmental plane to severing the intersegmental plane to achieve an oncologically safe surgical margin with no or minimal manual palpation and different landmarks. In this article, we present an overview of methods for each procedural step of thoracoscopic segmentectomy, from preoperative planning to division of the intersegmental plane.

Keywords

Thoracoscopy · Segmentectomy · Lung neoplasms · Simulation

H. E. Kim · Y. H. Yang · C. Y. Lee (✉)
Department of Thoracic and Cardiovascular Surgery, Severance Hospital, Yonsei University College of Medicine, Seoul, Republic of Korea
e-mail: cyleecs@yuhs.ac

3.1 Introduction

Lobectomy remains the gold-standard surgical treatment for primary lung cancer [1], but the frequency of thoracoscopic sublobar resection (SLR)—especially anatomical segmentectomy, which can achieve relatively secure and sufficient surgical margins—is increasing [2]. This phenomenon might be partially explained by the following reasons. First, with the popularization of low-dose computed tomography (CT), small lung cancers, such as ground-glasss opacity nodules (GGNs)—for which anatomical segmentectomy can achieve the same oncologic outcomes as lobectomy—have been detected more frequently. The characteristics of patients are also changing; physicians are more likely to encounter younger patients with small tumors for whom it is appropriate to consider a surgical extent that would spare lung parenchyma if a second cancer should develop [3]. Finally, there are increasingly many elderly patients with comorbidities in whom lung parenchyma should be preserved to reduce their postoperative morbidity and mortality [4]. In addition to primary lung cancer, segmentectomy can be performed for metastatic lung lesions or other non-malignant lung diseases, including inflammatory pseudotumors, congenital bronchial atresia, and pulmonary sequestration [5–9].

Relative to lobectomy, anatomical segmentectomy requires a thorough assessment of each patient's lung anatomy and a better understand-

K. Kim et al. (eds.), *Techniques in Minimally Invasive Thoracic Surgery*,
https://doi.org/10.1007/978-981-19-2472-9_3

ing of the branching patterns of the pulmonary vessels and bronchi [10]. In addition, numerous variations and anomalies of the pulmonary vessels and bronchus constitute issues to be overcome before performing segmentectomy. Although thoracoscopic segmentectomy has become a more common surgical procedure, surgeons should continue to be familiar with various methods, considering multiple factors such as the surgical margin, venous drainage of the tumor, and lung anatomy to conserve.

The purpose of this article was to present an overview of methods for each step of thoracoscopic segmentectomy, from preoperative planning to division of the intersegmental plane.

3.2 Preoperative Planning and Simulation

Segmentectomy is more complicated technically than lobectomy because of the anatomical complexity and variations of peripheral vessels and bronchi. Nagashima et al. [11, 12] and Shimizu et al. [13] reported that the prevalence of variations of bronchovascular patterns differed [14], sometimes significantly, from those noted by previous reports [15, 16]. In addition, unplanned procedures, such as additional wedge resection or completion lobectomy, are of concern during thoracoscopic segmentectomy [17]. Recently, three-dimensional (3D) imaging based on high-resolution CT has become more prevalent to help thoracic surgeons perform thoracoscopic segmentectomy by revealing the patient's anatomy in detail [18–22]. With this method, it is possible to: (1) specify the exact lesion location within a pulmonary segment, (2) define the segmental pulmonary artery or vein branches and bronchial tree divisions to identify possible anatomical variations, (3) calculate and integrate safety margins to prevent or decrease locoregional recurrence, (4) calculate the volume of the resected or nonresected segment, and (5) provide evidence to suggest alternative treatments in compromised patients for whom the 3D model was not suitable for anatomical segmentectomy due to anatomical or oncological reasons.

After our institution adopted a 3D workstation (SYNAPSE VINCENT: Fujifilm Medical, Tokyo, Japan) in October 2018, thin-section CT images were transferred to the 3D workstation to generate virtual 3D segmentectomy images. These simulation images were displayed on a monitor alongside the actual thoracoscopic monitor. For example, a female patient who presented with a persistent, 1.9-cm, part-solid GGN (ground-glass opacity percentage = 92%) on thin-section chest CT (Fig. 3.1a) was referred to our department and deemed suitable for SLR, with an adequate surgical margin. Although 3D reconstruction showed the safety margin (>60 mm) to be sufficient for upper-division segmentectomy, the remaining lung volume (28% of the left upper lobe [LUL] volume) was too small, suggesting insufficient preservation of the lung parenchyma (Fig. 3.1b). However, another 3D simulation (Fig. 3.1c) revealed that a safe surgical margin (37 mm) and preservation of lung parenchyma (74% of the LUL volume) could be simultaneously achieved when performing apicoposterior segmentectomy. Based on these results, apicoposterior segmentectomy was performed, and the parenchymal resection margin was measured as 3.0 cm on the pathologic examination.

However, it is important to interpret and utilize 3D models carefully in this context. Most importantly, the CT images and the consequent 3D model do not reflect lung collapse or deformity. Accordingly, the surgical margin from the 3D simulation is frequently overestimated relative to the gross or pathologic surgical margin [23].

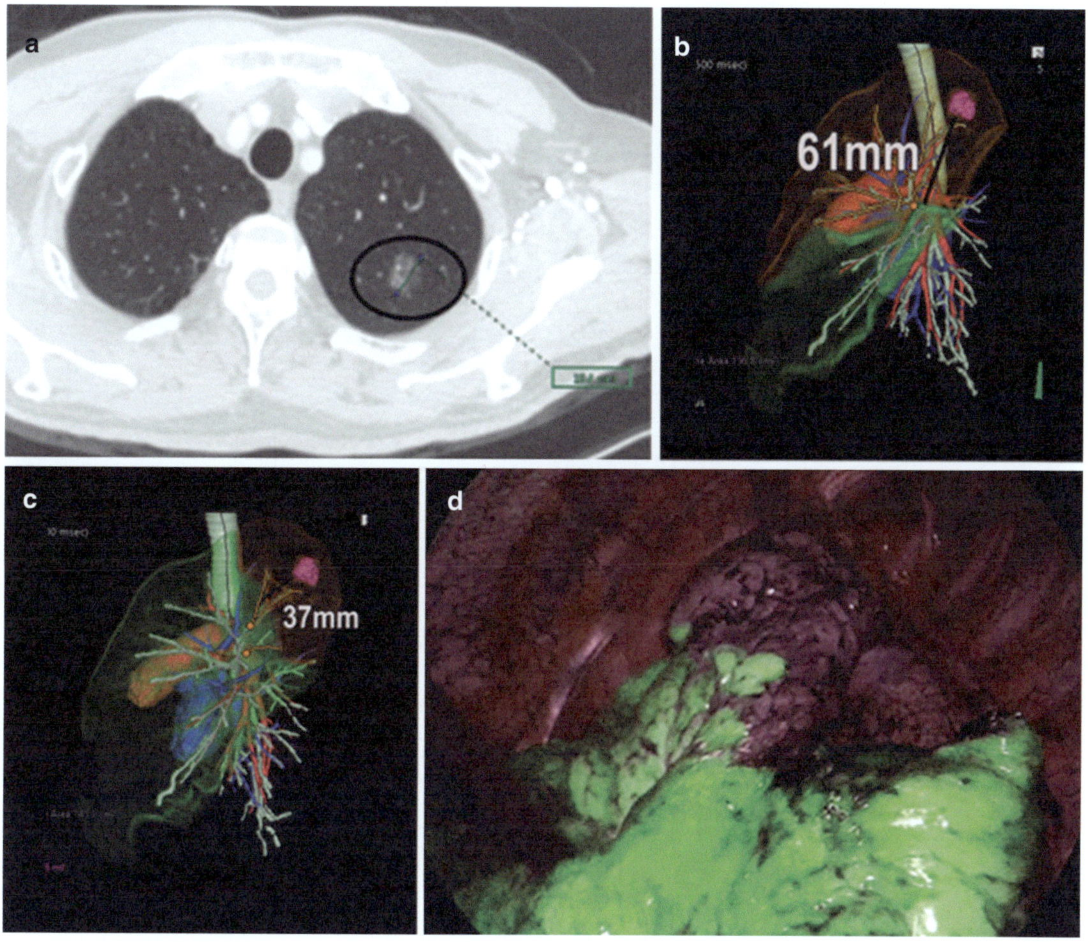

Fig. 3.1 (**a**) Axial view chest computed tomography (17-mm part-solid ground-glass nodule in the left upper lobe [LUL]). (**b**) A 3-dimensional (3D) simulation of left upper-division segmentectomy (virtual surgical margin: 61 mm, preserved lung volume: 392 mL [28% of the total LUL volume]). (**c**) A 3D simulation of left apicoposterior segmentectomy (virtual surgical margin: 37 mm, preserved lung volume: 1042 mL [74% of the total LUL volume]). (**d**) Corresponding surgical near-infrared thoracoscopy image after systemic indocyanine green injection

3.3 General Surgical Technique

Exposure of the Hilar Structures

The hilar structures should be exposed as much as possible to confirm the vascular or bronchial anatomy. For example, the left inferior pulmonary vein was dissected and exposed, as shown in Fig. 3.2a, when performing LS9, 10 segmentectomy from the posterior side; then, the segmental bronchus was exposed and grasped with atraumatic graspers (Fig. 3.2b). The lateral and back sides of the LS9, 10 segmental bronchi were dissected and isolated from the pulmonary artery branch with scissors or a tissue dissector (Fig. 3.2c) and divided with an endolinear stapler (Fig. 3.2d).

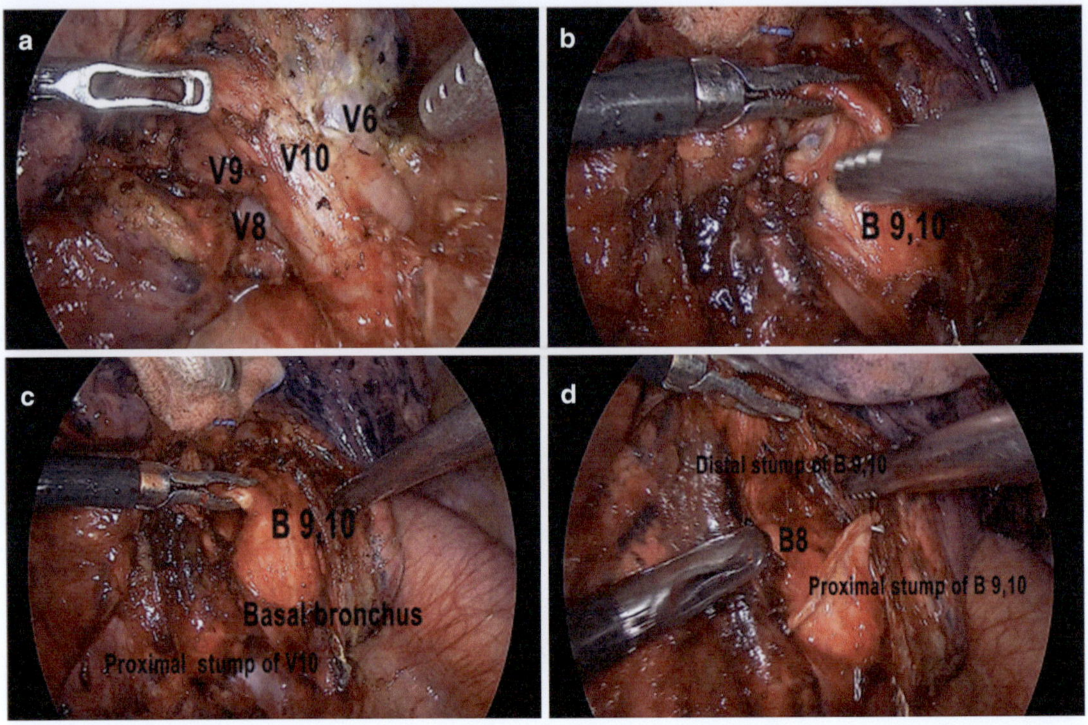

Fig. 3.2 (**a**) Full exposure of the left inferior pulmonary vein from the posterior side. (**b**) Grasping and lifting of the segmental bronchus. (**c**) Dissection of the lateral and posterior borders of the target bronchus. (**d**) Division and lifting of the distal stump of the target bronchus

Lifting the Distal Stump of the Vessels or Bronchus

Grasping and lifting the distal stump of the vessels or bronchus help to expose posterior segmental hilar structures [24]. For example, Fig. 3.3a shows that lifting distal V10 enabled easy exposure of B9, 10. In addition, grasping and further dissection of the resected bronchus help to expose and isolate the pulmonary artery branch (A10), as seen in Fig. 3.3b. Lifting the resected hilar structure also facilitates identification of the intersegmental vein branches and planes (Fig. 3.3c). Lastly, further dissection around resected hilar structures can make room for staplers (Fig. 3.3d). The technique is discussed in detail below.

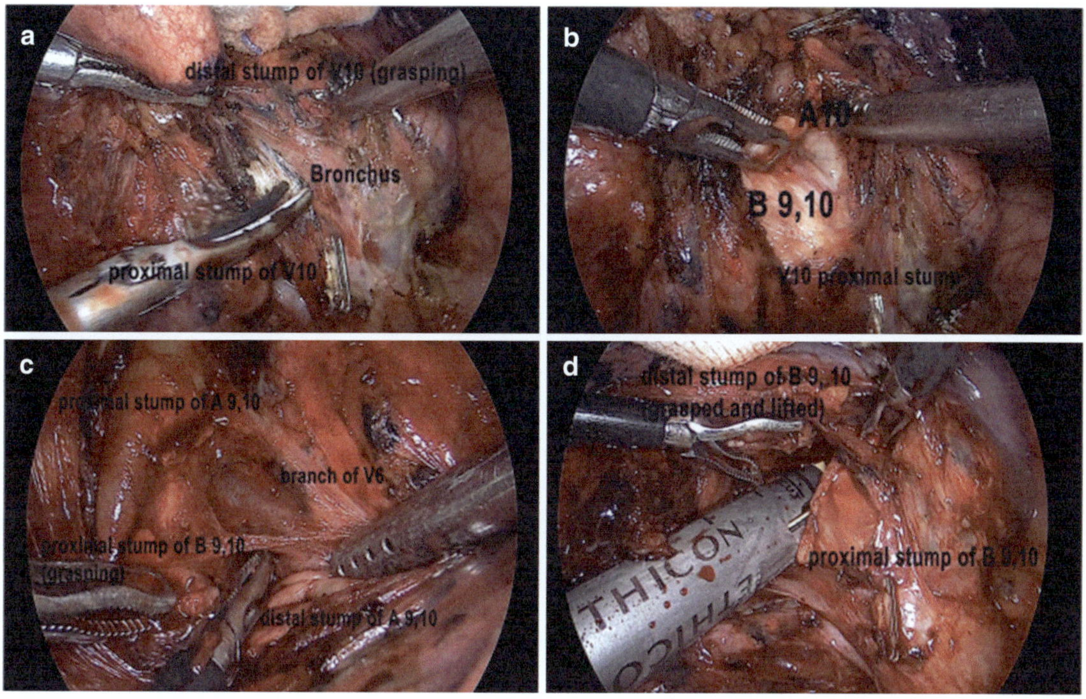

Fig. 3.3 (**a**) Lifting the distal stump of V10 to expose the target bronchus. (**b**) Grasping and lifting of B9, 10 to expose the posterior pulmonary artery. (**c**) Exposure of the intersegmental vein branch after division of A9, 10 and B9, 10. (**d**) Stapler insertion into the hilar pocket

3.4 Identification of the Intersegmental Plane

It is important to recognize and mark the intersegmental plane during anatomical segmentectomy. Several techniques have been introduced and established, as discussed below and summarized in Table 3.1.

Inflation–Deflation Method

Before dividing the clamped bronchus, the anesthesiologist is asked to ventilate the lung; thereafter, differential deflation and inflation of the segment to be removed are expected to develop, helping to delineate the intersegmental planes [25]. Although this is the most common method, its utility is less than satisfactory because the developing line is not as clear as desired due to collateral ventilation through Cohn's pores. Tsubota [26] reported using a method involving inflation of the whole lung; in this context, division of the segmental bronchus and opening of the stump of the preserved bronchus allowed the gas inside the preserved segments to escape. Okada et al. [27] suggested the utility of selective jet ventilation under flexible bronchoscopy in the segment to be resected. Other methods have been reported to inflate or keep the resected segment inflated, including bronchial ligation with a slipknot method after inflation or direct inflation by inserting a butterfly needle into the segmental bronchus [28, 29].

Perfusion Method

It is often difficult to delineate the intersegmental line in patients with emphysema using the inflation–deflation method because the lung parenchyma is likely to exhibit an advanced state of collateral respiratory structures, and inflated lungs typically hamper the surgical view during thora-

Table 3.1 Comparison of techniques to identify the intersegmental plane during thoracoscopic segmentectomy

Method	Inflation–deflation line		Intravenous indocyanine green	Virtual-assisted lung mapping
	Target segment deflated	Target segment inflated		
Advantages	– No preparation is necessary – Easy and quick	– Less interference with the surgical view – Relatively easy	– Easy and quick – Able to create the demarcation around the hilum	– Provides geometric information on the lung surface
Disadvantages	– Interference with the surgical view – Prolongation of the operation time – Intersegmental lines could be unclear due to collateral ventilation	– Some preparation or help of the anesthesiologist is needed – The needle injection method has been discarded due to air embolism – Intersegmental lines could be unclear due to collateral ventilation	– Correct identification of the pulmonary artery is necessary – An emphysematous lung that is less-perfused may be misleading or confusing – Infrared thoracoscopy is required	– Requires preoperative preparation – Basic instruments and some facilities are needed

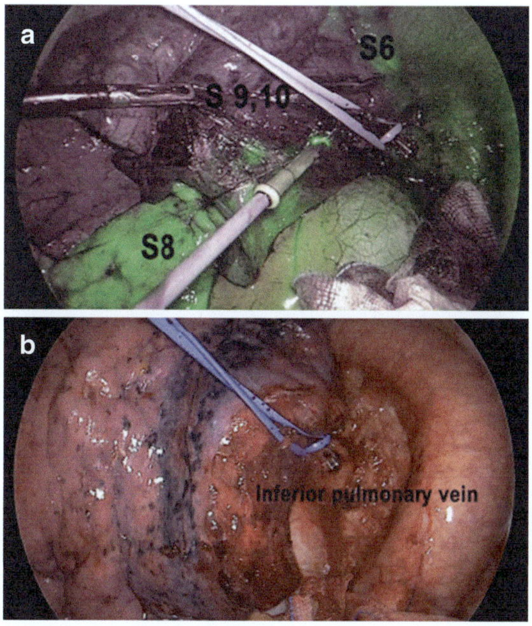

Fig. 3.4 (**a**) Demarcation of the intersegmental plane with electrocautery after systemic indocyanine green (ICG) injection. (**b**) Temporary pulmonary vein clamping to prevent ICG washout

coscopic segmentectomy, often resulting in delays in the procedure. To overcome these limitations of the inflation technique, Misaki et al. [30] introduced a novel method for visualizing adjacent segments using a near-infrared camera following systemic injection of indocyanine green (ICG). In this approach, after segmental pulmonary artery ligation or division, an intravenous injection of ICG creates a fluorescent demarcation between preserved (fluorescent) and targeted (nonfluorescent) segments (Fig. 3.4a) [31, 32]. However, it is often difficult to stain and dissect the correct intersegmental line within the few minutes before the ICG dye is washed out. However, Ito et al. [33] proposed a new technique in which the pulmonary vein of the entire lobe is clamped temporarily, prolonging ICG visualization (Fig. 3.4b).

Virtual-Assisted Pulmonary Mapping

This technique was developed as a bronchoscopic lung-marking method to avoid the inherent complications of CT-guided percutaneous lung marking. In virtual-assisted pulmonary mapping, multiple marks are made under the lung surface and provide geometric information for localizing a lesion in 3D space [34].

Division of the Intersegmental Plane

The optimal method for dissecting the intersegmental plane remains controversial. The two main approaches to developing the intersegmental plane involve using either stapling devices or energy instruments such as electrocautery or advanced bipolar energy. The use of energy devices has been considered advantageous for preserving pulmonary function due to the avoidance of squeezing or folding of the lungs by stapler devices [27]. However, it is possible that their use may lead to more postoperative complications, such as prolonged air leakage or bronchopleural fistula [35]. Recently, a randomized controlled trial reported a higher incidence of postoperative complications (e.g., air leakage) in the electrocautery group, while no difference was found in the loss of lung function [36]. However, there remain concerns that the effect of preserving lung function would be reduced by lung-folding involving multiple stapling actions when performing thoracoscopic complex segmentectomy. There are two main principles to follow to facilitate better inflation of preserved segments after thoracoscopic segmentectomy. First, the lung should be stapled from the periphery to the hilum. If multiple intersegmental planes need to be cut, peripheral stapling at different angles should be started and continued until reaching the center or hilum (Fig. 3.5a). Second, when the stapler reaches the hilum, it should be placed in the pocket (Fig. 3.5b) created by lifting the resected hilar structures as described above to involve the hilar structures of the target segment and to avoid cutting into the preserved segments. The cartilage, rather than the anvil of a stapler, should be placed toward the hilum to minimize the risk of vascular damage. Triangular (in a Mercedes-Benz mark-like fashion) (Fig. 3.5c) or V-shaped (or U-shaped) (Fig. 3.5d) stapling can be performed using these technical principles.

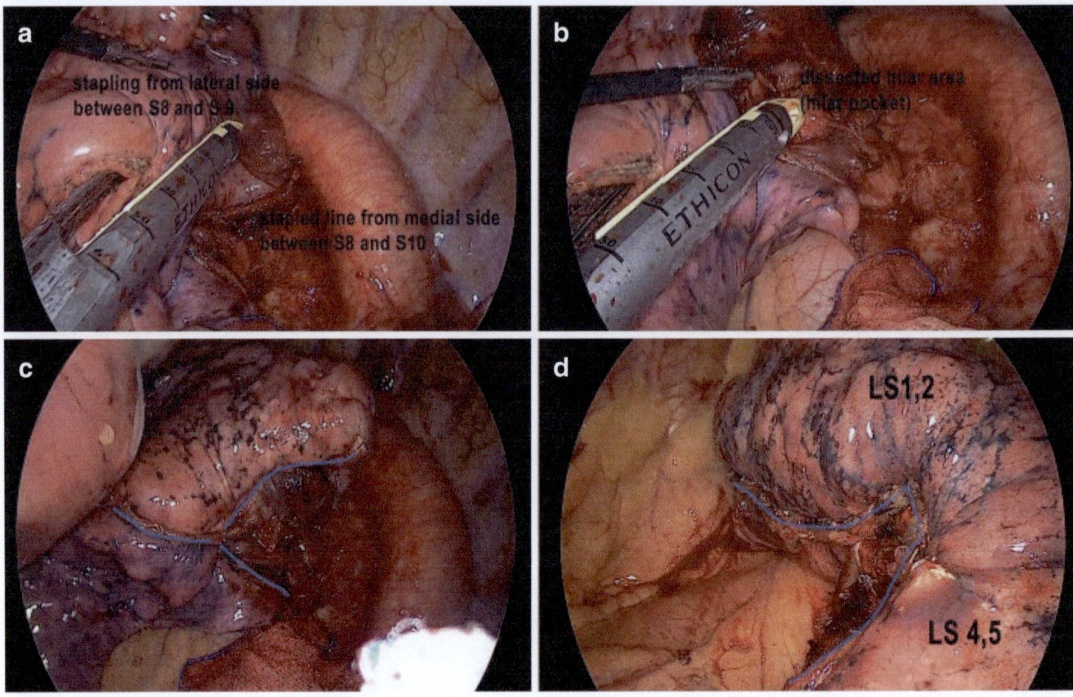

Fig. 3.5 (**a**) Peripheral stapling at different angles when starting the division of the intersegmental plane. (**b**) Placement of the stapler tip into the hilar pocket after further dissection of the hilar area. (**c**) Triangular stapled line after left 9, 10 segmentectomy. (**d**) A U-shaped (or V-shaped) stapled line after left 3 segmentectomy

3.5 Conclusion

Anatomical segmentectomy with thoracoscopy involves recognizing the correct 3D anatomy of the lung segment and accurately identifying the location of the lesion preoperatively or intraoperatively. Identifying and separating the intersegmental plane correctly and safely are important steps for completing thoracoscopic segmentectomy, with some technical pitfalls. In each step, different methods might be adopted based on the physician's preferences or situation. However, a thorough understanding of the advantages and limitations of each technique can help surgeons to perform lung segmentectomy more accurately.

Conflict of Interest No potential conflict of interest relevant to this article was reported.

References

1. Howington JA, Blum MG, Chang AC, Balekian AA, Murthy SC. Treatment of stage I and II non-small cell lung cancer: diagnosis and management of lung cancer, 3rd ed: American College of Chest Physicians evidence-based clinical practice guidelines. Chest. 2013;143(5 Suppl):e278S–313S.
2. Cao C, D'Amico T, Demmy T, et al. Less is more: a shift in the surgical approach to non-small-cell lung cancer. Lancet Respir Med. 2016;4:e11–2.
3. Gu C, Wang R, Pan X, et al. Sublobar resection versus lobectomy in patients aged ≤35 years with stage IA non-small cell lung cancer: a SEER database analysis. J Cancer Res Clin Oncol. 2017;143:2375–82.
4. Traibi A, Grigoroiu M, Boulitrop C, et al. Predictive factors for complications of anatomical pulmonary segmentectomies. Interact Cardiovasc Thorac Surg. 2013;17:838–44.
5. Shiono S, Okumura T, Boku N, et al. Outcomes of segmentectomy and wedge resection for pulmonary metastases from colorectal cancer. Eur J Cardiothorac Surg. 2017;51:504–10.

6. Berry MF. Role of segmentectomy for pulmonary metastases. Ann Cardiothorac Surg. 2014;3:176–82.
7. Melloni G, Carretta A, Ciriaco P, et al. Inflammatory pseudotumor of the lung in adults. Ann Thorac Surg. 2005;79:426–32.
8. Igai H, Kamiyoshihara M, Nagashima T, Shimizu K. Anatomical segmentectomy for pneumothorax associated with congenital bronchial atresia. Eur J Cardiothorac Surg. 2013;43:198.
9. Inoue T, Oizumi H, Nakamura M, Sadahiro M. Port-access thoracoscopic anatomical segmentectomy for pediatric intralobar pulmonary sequestration. Thorac Cardiovasc Surg Rep. 2014;3:42–4.
10. Shimizu K, Nakazawa S, Nagashima T, Kuwano H, Mogi A. 3D-CT anatomy for VATS segmentectomy. J Visc Surg. 2017;3:88.
11. Nagashima T, Shimizu K, Ohtaki Y, et al. An analysis of variations in the bronchovascular pattern of the right upper lobe using three-dimensional CT angiography and bronchography. Gen Thorac Cardiovasc Surg. 2015;63:354–60.
12. Nagashima T, Shimizu K, Ohtaki Y, et al. Analysis of variation in bronchovascular pattern of the right middle and lower lobes of the lung using three-dimensional CT angiography and bronchography. Gen Thorac Cardiovasc Surg. 2017;65:343–9.
13. Shimizu K, Nagashima T, Ohtaki Y, et al. Analysis of the variation pattern in right upper pulmonary veins and establishment of simplified vein models for anatomical segmentectomy. Gen Thorac Cardiovasc Surg. 2016;64:604–11.
14. Zhang M, Mao N, Zhang K, et al. Analysis of the variation pattern in left upper division veins and establishment of simplified vein models for anatomical segmentectomy. Ann Transl Med. 2020;8:1515.
15. Boyden EA, Scannell JG. An analysis of variations in the bronchovascular pattern of the right upper lobe of 50 lungs. Am J Anat. 1948;82:27–73.
16. Yamashita H. Variations in the pulmonary segments and the bronchovascular trees. In: Yamashita H, editor. Roentgenologic anatomy of the lung. Tokyo: Igaku-Shoin; 1978. p. 70–107.
17. Gossot D, Lutz JA, Grigoroiu M, Brian E, Seguin-Givelet A. Unplanned procedures during thoracoscopic segmentectomies. Ann Thorac Surg. 2017;104:1710–7.
18. Shimizu K, Nakano T, Kamiyoshihara M, Takeyoshi I. Segmentectomy guided by three-dimensional computed tomography angiography and bronchography. Interact Cardiovasc Thorac Surg. 2012;15:194–6.
19. Ikeda N, Yoshimura A, Hagiwara M, Akata S, Saji H. Three dimensional computed tomography lung modeling is useful in simulation and navigation of lung cancer surgery. Ann Thorac Cardiovasc Surg. 2013;19:1–5.
20. Akiba T. Utility of three-dimensional computed tomography in general thoracic surgery. Gen Thorac Cardiovasc Surg. 2013;61:676–84.
21. Oizumi H, Kanauchi N, Kato H, et al. Anatomic thoracoscopic pulmonary segmentectomy under 3-dimensional multidetector computed tomography simulation: a report of 52 consecutive cases. J Thorac Cardiovasc Surg. 2011;141:678–82.
22. Chen-Yoshikawa TF, Date H. Update on three-dimensional image reconstruction for preoperative simulation in thoracic surgery. J Thorac Dis. 2016;8(Suppl 3):S295–301.
23. Sato M, Murayama T, Nakajima J. Concepts and techniques: how to determine and identify the appropriate target segment in anatomical pulmonary segmentectomy? J Thorac Dis. 2019;11:972–86.
24. Sato M, Murayama T, Nakajima J. Techniques of stapler-based navigational thoracoscopic segmentectomy using virtual assisted lung mapping (VAL-MAP). J Thorac Dis. 2016;8(Suppl 9):S716–30.
25. Wells FC, Milstein BB. Thoracic surgical techniques. London: Bailliere Tindall; 1990. p. 126–34.
26. Tsubota N. An improved method for distinguishing the intersegmental plane of the lung. Surg Today. 2000;30:963–4.
27. Okada M, Mimura T, Ikegaki J, Katoh H, Itoh H, Tsubota N. A novel video-assisted anatomic segmentectomy technique: selective segmental inflation via bronchofiberoptic jet followed by cautery cutting. J Thorac Cardiovasc Surg. 2007;133:753–8.
28. Oizumi H, Kato H, Endoh M, Inoue T, Watarai H, Sadahiro M. Techniques to define segmental anatomy during segmentectomy. Ann Cardiothorac Surg. 2014;3:170–5.
29. Kamiyoshihara M, Kakegawa S, Morishita Y. Convenient and improved method to distinguish the intersegmental plane in pulmonary segmentectomy using a butterfly needle. Ann Thorac Surg. 2007;83:1913–4.
30. Misaki N, Chang SS, Gotoh M, Yamamoto Y, Satoh K, Yokomise H. A novel method for determining adjacent lung segments with infrared thoracoscopy. J Thorac Cardiovasc Surg. 2009;138:613–8.
31. Misaki N, Chang SS, Igai H, Tarumi S, Gotoh M, Yokomise H. New clinically applicable method for visualizing adjacent lung segments using an infrared thoracoscopy system. J Thorac Cardiovasc Surg. 2010;140:752–6.
32. Tarumi S, Misaki N, Kasai Y, Chang SS, Go T, Yokomise H. Clinical trial of video-assisted thoracoscopic segmentectomy using infrared thoracoscopy with indocyanine green. Eur J Cardiothorac Surg. 2014;46:112–5.
33. Ito A, Takao M, Shimamoto A, Shimpo H. Prolonged intravenous indocyanine green visualization by tem-

porary pulmonary vein clamping: real-time intraoperative fluorescence image guide for thoracoscopic anatomical segmentectomy. Eur J Cardiothorac Surg. 2017;52:1225–6.

34. Sato M, Kuwata T, Yamanashi K, et al. Safety and reproducibility of virtual-assisted lung mapping: a multicentre study in Japan. Eur J Cardiothorac Surg. 2017;51:861–8.

35. Ohtsuka T, Goto T, Anraku M, et al. Dissection of lung parenchyma using electrocautery is a safe and acceptable method for anatomical sublobar resection. J Cardiothorac Surg. 2012;7:42.

36. Chen X, Jin R, Xiang J, et al. Methods for dissecting intersegmental planes in segmentectomy: a randomized controlled trial. Ann Thorac Surg. 2020;110:258–64.

Video-Assisted Thoracic Surgery Lobectomy

4

Hong Kwan Kim

Abstract

Video-assisted thoracoscopic surgery (VATS) has been established as the surgical approach of choice for lobectomy in patients with early-stage non-small cell lung cancer (NSCLC). Patients with clinical stage I NSCLC with no lymph node metastasis are considered candidates for VATS lobectomy. To rule out the presence of metastasis to lymph nodes or distant organs, patients should undergo meticulous clinical staging. Assessing patients' functional status is required to ensure that there are no medical contraindications, such as impaired pulmonary function or cardiac comorbidities. Although various combinations of the number, size, and location of ports are available, finding the best method of port placement for each surgeon is fundamental to maximize the efficiency of the surgical procedure. When conducting VATS lobectomy, it is always necessary to comply with the following oncological principles: (1) the vessels and bronchus of the target lobe should be individually divided, (2) systematic lymph node dissection is mandatory, and (3) touching the lymph node itself and rupturing the capsule of the lymph node should be minimized. Most surgeons conduct the procedure in the following sequence: (1) dissection along the hilar structure, (2) fissure division, (3) perivascular and peribronchial dissection, (4) individual division of the vessels and bronchus, (5) specimen retrieval, and (6) mediastinal lymph node dissection. Surgeons should obtain experience in enhancing the exposure of the dissection target and facilitating dissection. This review article provides the basic principles of the surgical techniques and practical maneuvers for performing VATS lobectomy easily, safely, and efficiently.

Keywords

Lung neoplasms · Video-assisted thoracic surgery · Lobectomy

4.1 Introduction

During the past three decades, video-assisted thoracoscopic surgery (VATS) has been established as the gold-standard surgical approach for lobectomy in patients with early-stage non-small cell lung cancer (NSCLC). Due to the tremendous efforts of pioneers in this field [1–7], thoracic surgeons have been increasingly adopting VATS lobectomy [8, 9]. Evidence has accumulated that the early and late outcomes of VATS are comparable or even superior to those of open thoracot-

H. K. Kim (✉)
Department of Thoracic and Cardiovascular Surgery, Samsung Medical Center, Sungkyunkwan University School of Medicine, Seoul, Republic of Korea
e-mail: hkts.kim@samsung.com

K. Kim et al. (eds.), *Techniques in Minimally Invasive Thoracic Surgery*,
https://doi.org/10.1007/978-981-19-2472-9_4

omy [1–17]. Several recent large-scale database analyses have shown that VATS lobectomy can be conducted with improved short-term outcomes [18–25] and favorable long-term survival compared with open thoracotomy lobectomy [26]. Therefore, VATS lobectomy is now strongly recommended for patients without surgical and medical contraindications unless the oncological principles of surgery are compromised. This review article provides the basic principles of the surgical techniques and practical maneuvers for performing VATS lobectomy easily, safely, and efficiently.

4.2 Definition and Indications

Despite various modifications in the surgical techniques of VATS lobectomy, the most widely accepted definition was established by the CALGB 39082 trial as a procedure including a 4- to 8-cm access incision and a totally endoscopic approach, without rib spreading and individual anatomical dissection and division of the pulmonary vein, artery, and bronchus [7].

The most important prerequisite of successful VATS lobectomy is to select optimal patients with tumor features suitable for a minimally invasive surgical approach. Conventionally, most patients with clinical stage I NSCLC without lymph node metastasis can be considered candidates for VATS lobectomy. However, the tumor/node/metastasis classification system by the American Joint Committee on Cancer has been updated to the eighth edition, where tumors larger than 4 cm and 5 cm without nodal involvement are classified as stage IIA and IIB, respectively. Therefore, even clinical stage IIA or IIB NSCLC tumors classified using the tumor size criterion can be considered as candidates for VATS lobectomy as long as no nodal or distant organ metastases are present. Nonetheless, debate continues regarding the size barrier at which the VATS approach is discouraged. Although some surgeons argue that tumors larger than 7 cm, which are classified as stage T4 or IIIA, can be safely and effectively removed using the VATS approach, an issue exists regarding whether oncological principles can be satisfied with this minimally invasive approach for such large tumors that show biological aggressiveness [27]. The most commonly used size limit is 6–7 cm. Alternatively, many investigators have attempted to expand the indication of VATS lobectomy. Some adopted the VATS approach for node-positive NSCLC, and others have tried it after neoadjuvant therapy [28–37]. We should be cautious when extending the indications of the VATS approach since it could lead to an increased risk of procedure-related recurrence due to the possibility of cancer dissemination during VATS manipulation, the risk of leaving residual tumors at the surgical margin, and the apprehension of performing insufficient lymph node dissection [11].

4.3 Patient Assessment and Preparation

To rule out metastasis to lymph nodes or distant organs, patients should undergo meticulous clinical staging. Staging workups include computed tomography (CT) of the chest and upper abdomen and positron emission tomography–CT with 18F-fluorodeoxyglucose. When these tests suggest mediastinal nodal metastasis, patients should be evaluated using mediastinoscopy. However, mediastinoscopy has recently been replaced with less invasive procedures, such as endobronchial and/or endoscopic ultrasonography, and then transbronchial or transesophageal needle aspiration biopsy is performed for histological confirmation. Brain magnetic resonance imaging is needed to assess the presence of brain metastasis, especially if patients have headaches or neurological symptoms. Bronchoscopy should be performed to evaluate the presence of endobronchial lesions in patients with centrally located tumors.

Apart from the tumor characteristics, assessing patients' functional status is required to ensure that no medical contraindications exist, such as impaired pulmonary function or cardiac comorbidities. Baseline pulmonary function is assessed using spirometry, and echocardiography can be performed to assess baseline cardiac function. The essential component for predicting preoperative and postoperative pulmonary function is forced expiratory volume in 1 s (FEV1). More importantly, the diffusing capacity of carbon monoxide (DLco) is critical for predicting the risk of postoperative pulmonary complications. When the postoperative FEV1 or DLco measurement is less than 40% of the predicted value, surgery should be declined, regardless of whether the VATS approach is used [38]. When the predicted postoperative FEV1 or DLco value is marginal (i.e., 40–60%), suggesting a moderate risk of postoperative pulmonary complications, patients should be further evaluated using exercise tests, such as the 6-min walk test or oxygen consumption test [38, 39].

4.4 General Anesthesia and Positioning

Single-lung ventilation using a double-lumen endotracheal tube is mandatory to achieve an excellent surgical exposure and operative view. The anesthesiologist should ensure that the double-lumen endotracheal tube is in the correct position, and then ventilation can be maintained only in the contralateral lung to optimize deflation of the ipsilateral lung. If the lung does not effectively deflate, suction is occasionally applied. The respiratory rate can be increased to 20 breaths/min or more to achieve a more stable operative view since a decrease in the tidal volume by increasing the respiratory rate could reduce the degree of mediastinal deviation due to ventilation. During single-lung ventilation, maintaining adequate oxygenation is difficult even in patients with preserved pulmonary function because a ventilation–perfusion mismatch intrinsically occurs due to continuous perfusion to the non-ventilated lung. Whenever hypoxia occurs, temporarily pausing the procedure and then permitting double-lung ventilation until the hypoxic state is corrected would be better. Otherwise, anesthesiologists tend to apply high-pressure ventilation to the contralateral lung under single-lung ventilation, which would in turn put the patient at a higher risk of postoperative lung injury.

Following the induction of single-lung ventilation and general anesthesia, the patient is placed in the lateral decubitus position. The hands are placed unsupported in the "prayer" position in front of the face. The operating table is adjusted to flex the patient adequately to maximize intercostal space widening. During this maneuver, care should be taken not to overextend the shoulder and elbow, which could result in brachial plexus injury. Since changing the patient's position could cause the double-lumen endotracheal tube to deviate from the proper position, the anesthesiologist should recheck the placement of the endotracheal tube immediately after the patient is rotated into the lateral decubitus position. The position of the surgeon depends on the surgeon's preferences for the surgical approach and port placement.

4.5 Port Placement

Various port placement options have been devised and modified by several surgeons. With adequate port placement, the surgical procedure can be smooth and easy. However, if port placement is inadequate, easy cases might become technically challenging, which might adversely affect the degree to which the procedure follows oncological principles. Therefore, finding an effective method of port placement that best fits and is comfortable for each surgeon is fundamental to maximize the efficiency of the surgical procedure. Various combinations of the number, size, and location of ports are available. Conventionally, a 4- to 5-cm utility incision accompanied by a 5- to 10-mm port for the thoracoscope and a 5-mm additional port for left-hand instruments is made [12]. The location of the ports depends on the surgical approach (anterior versus posterior) and thoracoscopic view (conventional panoramic view versus direct hilar view) (Fig. 4.1). Some pioneers in the field have recently attempted to reduce the number of ports, and uniportal or biportal VATS lobectomy is now widely adopted by several surgeons [40, 41].

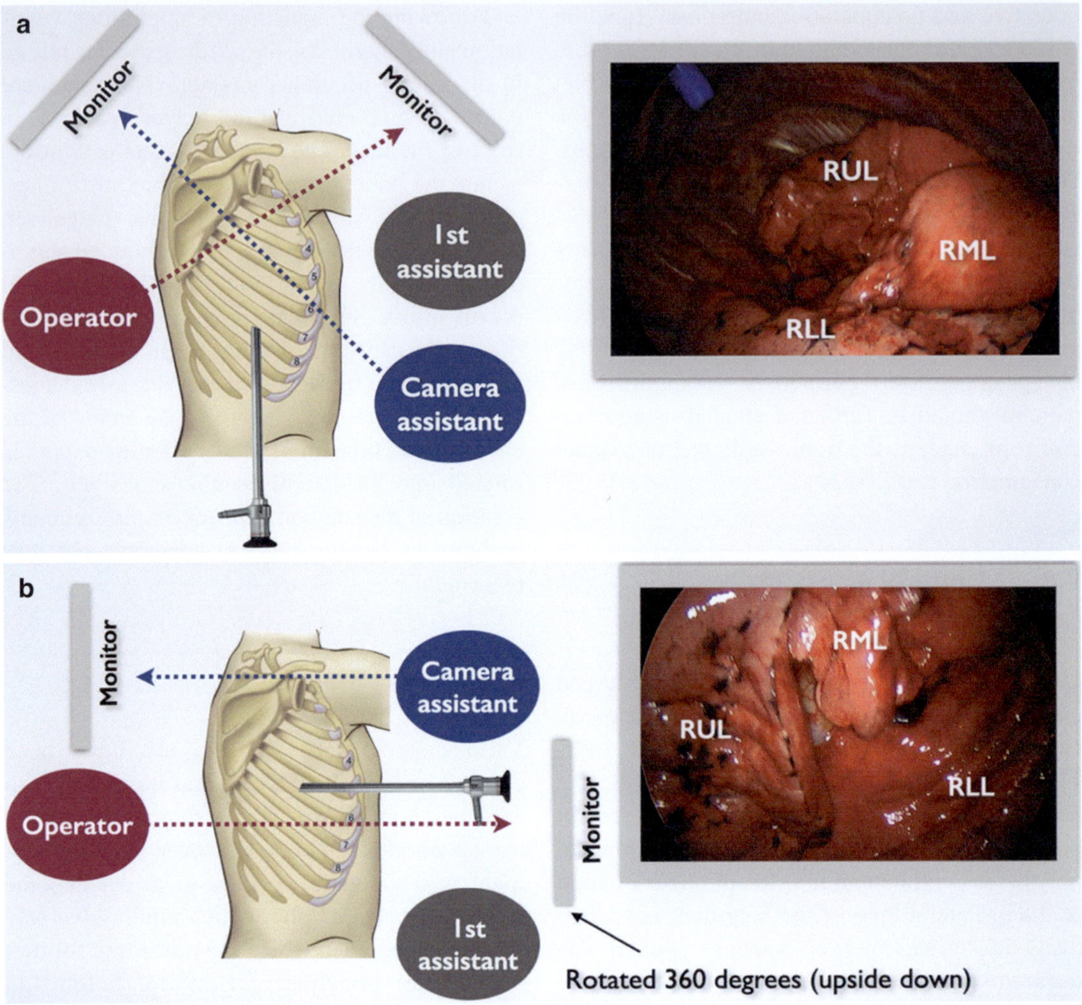

Fig. 4.1 The location of the ports depends on the thoracoscopic view. (**a**) Conventional panoramic view. (**b**) Direct hilar view. *RUL* right upper lobe, *RML* right middle lobe

4.6 Main Procedure

Despite these technical variations, especially in port placement, the following oncological principles should always be complied with: (1) the vessels and bronchus of the target lobe should be individually divided, (2) systematic lymph node dissection is mandatory, and (3) touching the lymph node itself and rupturing the capsule of the lymph node should be minimized. Although there could be modifications, most surgeons conduct the procedure in the following sequence: (1) dissection along the hilar structure, (2) fissure division, (3) perivascular and peribronchial dissection, (4) individual division of the vessels and bronchus, (5) specimen retrieval, and (6) mediastinal lymph node dissection. Although some anatomical variations could exist according to the target lobe to be resected in VATS lobectomy, the general principles of dissection techniques along the hilar structure and perivascular/peribronchial space are the same across the target lobes. In principle, surgeons should obtain experience in enhancing the exposure of the dissection target and facilitating the dissection.

The anterior surface of the vessel is usually easy to dissect since we can see it directly, whereas the posterior surface of the vessel is difficult to dissect because achieving direct exposure is difficult. Therefore, to enhance the exposure, especially in the posterior surface of the vascular structure, critical maneuvers should be kept in mind. For example, gently grasping the target vessel with soft-surfaced endoscopic forceps or graspers could provide better exposure of the area behind the structure (Fig. 4.2). Considering that the pulmonary artery is easier to tear or injure than the pulmonary vein, special care should be taken when grasping the pulmonary artery. For this maneuver, we can imagine how a lioness never hurts her cub if she gently holds it with her sharp teeth. Another method to enhance the exposure of the posterior area is to lift the vessel using various instruments, such as graspers, an electrocautery tip, and a suction device. After clearing the soft tissue around the anterior and posterior surfaces of the target vessel, instruments (e.g., a right-angled clamp and endoscopic stapler) can be easily and safely passed along.

Several useful methods exist to facilitate hilar and perivascular dissection, including bimanual dissection, holding the shaft of the instruments short, digging or tunneling, and spreading. First, for effective dissection, coordinating 2 hands is crucial. If the surgeon uses only 1 hand, dissection will become more difficult and unsafe. Unless the surgeon has only 1 hand, the dissection will be more effective if the surgeon takes advantage of the non-dominant hand (the left hand if one is right-handed and vice versa).

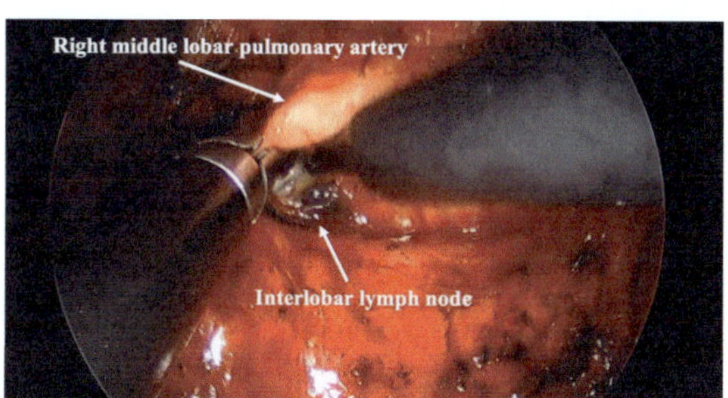

Fig. 4.2 Gentle grasping of the pulmonary artery using an instrument. Gently grasping the target vessel with soft-surfaced endoscopic forceps or graspers could provide better exposure of the area behind the structure

Constant practice in daily life is necessary to get used to using one's non-dominant hand. Second, it feels unexpectedly effective if one holds the shaft of every instrument, not its handle. In the VATS procedure, a fulcrum effect always occurs since there is a long distance between the port entrance and the target structure. If one holds the instrument rather short or even in the middle, the fulcrum is shortened, and then the dissection process becomes much easier (Fig. 4.3). Third, if the surgeon identifies the appropriate plane after the initial dissection, further dissection can be easily conducted, as if he or she is digging or tunneling using two instruments of both hands. In the same context, one can make the dissection safer and more effective by spreading out the jaws of the graspers. Finally, it is crucial to keep in mind the principle that one should conduct peribronchial dissection rather than perivascular dissection every time one dissects a vessel. If one focuses on perivascular dissection too much, dissection could be more difficult and dangerous since it is possible to denude the surface of the vessel, especially in elderly patients with fragile vascular walls. Alternatively, if one simply focuses on peribronchial dissection, not perivascular dissection, and then assesses the lymph nodes around the bronchus, one might eventually realize that perivascular dissection is conducted after completing the peribronchial dissection.

Although VATS lobectomy is easy to perform in cases of complete interlobar fissure, partially complete or totally incomplete fissures are often identified. For partially complete fissures, bidirectionally dissecting the plane is helpful. Imagine the situation of playing around the seashore as a child making a sand tunnel. During this activity, we carefully dissect the sand in one way first and then in the opposite way, not to destroy the tunnel. As with the sand tunnel, it will be much safer if one completely dissects around the surrounding structure bidirectionally before encircling the fissure and even any vital structures. However, for totally incomplete fissures, adopting a completely different approach is necessary, such as the fissureless technique or the hilar-first technique [42]. In this situation, one must dissect the hilar structure first and then

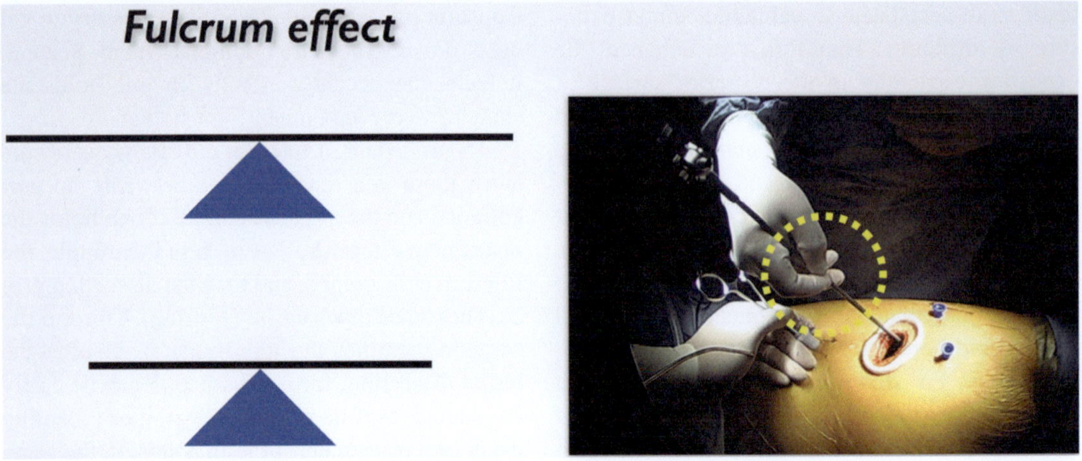

Fig. 4.3 One should hold the shaft of the instrument short to reduce the fulcrum effect. If one holds the instrument rather short or even in the middle, the fulcrum is also shortened, and the dissection process then becomes much easier

divide the pulmonary vein and arteries, followed by the bronchus, and divide the fissure last. Before one attempts this technique, it is crucial to gain experience through practice and to reach a complete understanding of the anatomy.

Conventionally, the sequence of the division of bronchovascular structures is as follows: pulmonary vein, pulmonary artery, and then the lobar bronchus. Theoretically, the pulmonary-vein-first technique prevents tumor cells from spreading into the systemic circulation, which could result from surgical manipulation, whereas the pulmonary-artery-first technique can cause tumor cells to spread into the systemic circulation via the intact pulmonary vein [43]. Some investigators have shown that the ligation of the pulmonary vein first during surgery may help prevent blood micro-metastases [44]. However, in another randomized controlled trial comparing long-term survival according to the sequence of pulmonary vessel ligation, no significant differences were found between the two groups [45]. Conversely, early division of the pulmonary vein can cause venous congestion of the target lobe, leading to difficulties in exposure, manipulation, and specimen removal after the main procedure. However, there is still no consensus regarding the sequence of the division of the vascular structures, and further studies should be conducted before drawing firm conclusions.

4.7 Conclusion

As minimally invasive techniques, such as the VATS approach, have been introduced into the field of surgical treatment of lung cancer, patients have been able to benefit from less invasive surgical approaches with lower morbidity and higher recovery, without compromising oncological outcomes. Nonetheless, the VATS approach is only a method for surgically treating patients, not a purpose per se. Assessing the indications for VATS lobectomy and preparing patients before surgery are crucial for obtaining excellent outcomes. To conduct VATS lobectomy safely and effectively, it is of fundamental importance to keep in mind the principles of the procedure and to practice the procedure regularly.

Conflict of Interest No potential conflict of interest relevant to this article was reported.

References

1. Kirby TJ, Mack MJ, Landreneau RJ, Rice TW. Lobectomy: video-assisted thoracic surgery versus muscle-sparing thoracotomy: a randomized trial. J Thorac Cardiovasc Surg. 1995;109:997–1002.
2. Sugi K, Kaneda Y, Esato K. Video-assisted thoracoscopic lobectomy achieves a satisfactory long-term prognosis in patients with clinical stage IA lung cancer. World J Surg. 2000;24:27–31.

3. McKenna RJ Jr, Houck W, Fuller CB. Video-assisted thoracic surgery lobectomy: experience with 1100 cases. Ann Thorac Surg. 2006;81:421–6.
4. Onaitis MW, Petersen RP, Balderson SS, et al. Thoracoscopic lobectomy is a safe and versatile procedure: experience with 500 consecutive patients. Ann Surg. 2006;244:420–5.
5. Shigemura N, Akashi A, Funaki S, et al. Long-term outcomes after a variety of video-assisted thoracoscopic lobectomy approaches for clinical stage IA lung cancer: a multi-institutional study. J Thorac Cardiovasc Surg. 2006;132:507–12.
6. Mun M, Kohno T. Efficacy of thoracoscopic resection for multifocal bronchioloalveolar carcinoma showing pure ground-glass opacities of 20 mm or less in diameter. J Thorac Cardiovasc Surg. 2007;134:877–82.
7. Swanson SJ, Herndon JE 2nd, D'Amico TA, et al. Video-assisted thoracic surgery lobectomy: report of CALGB 39802: a prospective, multi-institution feasibility study. J Clin Oncol. 2007;25:4993–7.
8. Whitson BA, Andrade RS, Boettcher A, et al. Video-assisted thoracoscopic surgery is more favorable than thoracotomy for resection of clinical stage I non-small cell lung cancer. Ann Thorac Surg. 2007;83:1965–70.
9. Flores RM, Park BJ, Dycoco J, et al. Lobectomy by video-assisted thoracic surgery (VATS) versus thoracotomy for lung cancer. J Thorac Cardiovasc Surg. 2009;138:11–8.
10. Villamizar NR, Darrabie MD, Burfeind WR, et al. Thoracoscopic lobectomy is associated with lower morbidity compared with thoracotomy. J Thorac Cardiovasc Surg. 2009;138:419–25.
11. Yan TD, Black D, Bannon PG, McCaughan BC. Systematic review and meta-analysis of randomized and nonrandomized trials on safety and efficacy of video-assisted thoracic surgery lobectomy for early-stage non-small-cell lung cancer. J Clin Oncol. 2009;27:2553–62.
12. Kim K, Kim HK, Park JS, et al. Video-assisted thoracic surgery lobectomy: single institutional experience with 704 cases. Ann Thorac Surg. 2010;89:S2118–22.
13. Scott WJ, Allen MS, Darling G, et al. Video-assisted thoracic surgery versus open lobectomy for lung cancer: a secondary analysis of data from the American College of Surgeons Oncology Group Z0030 randomized clinical trial. J Thorac Cardiovasc Surg. 2010;139:976–83.
14. D'Amico TA, Niland J, Mamet R, Zornosa C, Dexter EU, Onaitis MW. Efficacy of mediastinal lymph node dissection during lobectomy for lung cancer by thoracoscopy and thoracotomy. Ann Thorac Surg. 2011;92:226–32.
15. Hanna WC, de Valence M, Atenafu EG, et al. Is video-assisted lobectomy for non-small-cell lung cancer oncologically equivalent to open lobectomy? Eur J Cardiothorac Surg. 2013;43:1121–5.
16. Kuritzky AM, Aswad BI, Jones RN, Ng T. Lobectomy by video-assisted thoracic surgery vs muscle-sparing thoracotomy for stage I lung cancer: a critical evaluation of short- and long-term outcomes. J Am Coll Surg. 2015;220:1044–53.
17. Mei J, Guo C, Xia L, et al. Long-term survival outcomes of video-assisted thoracic surgery lobectomy for stage I–II non-small cell lung cancer are more favorable than thoracotomy: a propensity score-matched analysis from a high-volume center in China. Transl Lung Cancer Res. 2019;8:155–66.
18. Paul S, Altorki NK, Sheng S, et al. Thoracoscopic lobectomy is associated with lower morbidity than open lobectomy: a propensity-matched analysis from the STS database. J Thorac Cardiovasc Surg. 2010;139:366–78.
19. Paul S, Sedrakyan A, Chiu YL, et al. Outcomes after lobectomy using thoracoscopy vs thoracotomy: a comparative effectiveness analysis utilizing the Nationwide Inpatient Sample database. Eur J Cardiothorac Surg. 2013;43:813–7.
20. Boffa DJ, Dhamija A, Kosinski AS, et al. Fewer complications result from a video-assisted approach to anatomic resection of clinical stage I lung cancer. J Thorac Cardiovasc Surg. 2014;148:637–43.
21. Paul S, Isaacs AJ, Treasure T, Altorki NK, Sedrakyan A. Long term survival with thoracoscopic versus open lobectomy: propensity matched comparative analysis using SEER-Medicare database. BMJ. 2014;349:g5575.
22. Falcoz PE, Puyraveau M, Thomas PA, et al. Video-assisted thoracoscopic surgery versus open lobectomy for primary non-small-cell lung cancer: a propensity-matched analysis of outcome from the European Society of Thoracic Surgeon database. Eur J Cardiothorac Surg. 2016;49:602–9.
23. Laursen LO, Petersen RH, Hansen HJ, Jensen TK, Ravn J, Konge L. Video-assisted thoracoscopic surgery lobectomy for lung cancer is associated with a lower 30-day morbidity compared with lobectomy by thoracotomy. Eur J Cardiothorac Surg. 2016;49:870–5.
24. Medbery RL, Gillespie TW, Liu Y, et al. Nodal upstaging is more common with thoracotomy than with VATS during lobectomy for early-stage lung cancer: an analysis from the National Cancer Data Base. J Thorac Oncol. 2016;11:222–33.
25. Pages PB, Delpy JP, Orsini B, et al. Propensity score analysis comparing videothoracoscopic lobectomy with thoracotomy: a French nationwide study. Ann Thorac Surg. 2016;101:1370–8.
26. Yang CJ, Kumar A, Klapper JA, et al. A national analysis of long-term survival following thoracoscopic versus open lobectomy for stage I non-small-cell lung cancer. Ann Surg. 2019;269:163–71.
27. Yan TD, Cao C, D'Amico TA, et al. Video-assisted thoracoscopic surgery lobectomy at 20 years: a consensus statement. Eur J Cardiothorac Surg. 2014;45:633–9.
28. Dell'Amore A, Lomangino I, Tamburini N, et al. Video-assisted thoracoscopic lobectomy after neoadjuvant chemotherapy for non-small cell lung cancer: a

multicenter propensity-matched study. Surg Endosc. 2021;36(2):1466–75. https://doi.org/10.1007/s00464-021-08431-z.
29. Deng HY, Qiu XM, Zhu DX, Tang X, Zhou Q. Video-assisted thoracoscopic sleeve lobectomy for centrally located non-small cell lung cancer: a meta-analysis. World J Surg. 2021;45:897–906.
30. Gao HJ, Jiang ZH, Gong L, et al. Video-assisted vs thoracotomy sleeve lobectomy for lung cancer: a propensity matched analysis. Ann Thorac Surg. 2019;108:1072–9.
31. Kamel MK, Nasar A, Stiles BM, Altorki NK, Port JL. Video-assisted thoracoscopic lobectomy is the preferred approach following induction chemotherapy. J Laparoendosc Adv Surg Tech A. 2017;27:495–500.
32. Kim HK, Choi YS, Kim J, Shim YM, Kim K. Outcomes of unexpected pathologic N1 and N2 disease after video-assisted thoracic surgery lobectomy for clinical stage I non-small cell lung cancer. J Thorac Cardiovasc Surg. 2010;140:1288–93.
33. Romero Roman A, Campo-Canaveral de la Cruz JL, Macia I, et al. Outcomes of surgical resection after neoadjuvant chemoimmunotherapy in locally advanced stage IIIA non-small-cell lung cancer. Eur J Cardiothorac Surg. 2021;60:81–8.
34. Xie D, Zhong Y, Deng J, et al. Comparison of uniportal video-assisted thoracoscopic versus thoracotomy bronchial sleeve lobectomy with pulmonary arterioplasty for centrally located non-small-cell lung cancer. Eur J Cardiothorac Surg. 2021;59:978–86.
35. Yang CF, Meyerhoff RR, Mayne NR, et al. Long-term survival following open versus thoracoscopic lobectomy after preoperative chemotherapy for non-small cell lung cancer. Eur J Cardiothorac Surg. 2016;49:1615–23.
36. Yun JK, Lee GD, Choi S, et al. Video-assisted thoracoscopic lobectomy is feasible for selected patients with clinical N2 non-small cell lung cancer. Sci Rep. 2020;10:15217.
37. Yun JK, Park I, Kim HR, et al. Long-term outcomes of video-assisted thoracoscopic lobectomy for clinical N1 non-small cell lung cancer: a propensity score-weighted comparison with open thoracotomy. Lung Cancer. 2020;150:201–8.
38. Postmus PE, Kerr KM, Oudkerk M, et al. Early and locally advanced non-small-cell lung cancer (NSCLC): ESMO Clinical Practice Guidelines for diagnosis, treatment and follow-up. Ann Oncol. 2017;28(suppl_4):41–21.
39. Lee H, Kim HK, Kang D, et al. Prognostic value of 6-min walk test to predict postoperative cardiopulmonary complications in patients with non-small cell lung cancer. Chest. 2020;157:1665–73.
40. Gonzalez-Rivas D, Paradela M, Fieira E, Velasco C. Single-incision video-assisted thoracoscopic lobectomy: initial results. J Thorac Cardiovasc Surg. 2012;143:745–7.
41. Rocco G, Martin-Ucar A, Passera E. Uniportal VATS wedge pulmonary resections. Ann Thorac Surg. 2004;77:726–8.
42. Decaluwe H, Sokolow Y, Deryck F, et al. Thoracoscopic tunnel technique for anatomical lung resections: a 'fissure first, hilum last' approach with staplers in the fissureless patient. Interact Cardiovasc Thorac Surg. 2015;21:2–7.
43. Wei S, Guo C, He J, et al. Effect of vein-first vs artery-first surgical technique on circulating tumor cells and survival in patients with non-small cell lung cancer: a randomized clinical trial and registry-based propensity score matching analysis. JAMA Surg. 2019;154:e190972.
44. Song PP, Zhang W, Zhang B, Liu Q, DU J. Effects of different sequences of pulmonary artery and vein ligations during pulmonary lobectomy on blood micrometastasis of non-small cell lung cancer. Oncol Lett. 2013;5:463–8.
45. Kozak A, Alchimowicz J, Safranow K, et al. The impact of the sequence of pulmonary vessel ligation during anatomic resection for lung cancer on long-term survival: a prospective randomized trial. Adv Med Sci. 2013;58:156–63.

Video-Assisted Thoracic Surgery Bronchial Sleeve Lobectomy

5

Hyeong Ryul Kim

Abstract

Sleeve lobectomy is performed to preserve lung function in patients with central lung cancer. Recent advances in surgical skill can make this complex procedure possible with video-assisted thoracic surgery (VATS). VATS sleeve lobectomy is technically challenging; however, it can be safely performed by an experienced surgeon.

5.1 Introduction

Bronchial sleeve resection is a complex procedure comprising bronchial resection and end-to-end anastomosis. Sleeve lobectomy was first described in 1947 by Clement Price Thomas [1, 2] and was widely adopted to resect tumors invading the central lung while conserving pulmonary function [3, 4]. More recently, as surgeons have obtained experience with video-assisted thoracoscopic surgery (VATS), complex procedures such as tracheal and bronchial/vascular sleeve resection have been attempted thoracoscopically [5, 6]. We describe the surgical skills involved in thoracoscopic bronchial sleeve lobectomy.

H. R. Kim (✉)
Department of Thoracic and Cardiovascular Surgery, Asan Medical Center, University of Ulsan College of Medicine, Seoul, Republic of Korea
e-mail: hrkim09@ulsan.ac.kr

5.2 Methods

Anesthesia

After the patient receives an intravenous bolus of muscle relaxant and short-acting anesthetic agents, general anesthesia is induced with double-lumen endotracheal intubation. The anesthesiologist uses a flexible bronchoscope to check the location of the endotracheal tube. Anesthesia is maintained by either volatile or intravenous anesthetic agents. An opioid is administered continuously during surgery; to adjust the dosage, the anesthesiologist assesses hemodynamic parameters. Patients are ventilated to achieve normocapnia (35–45 mmHg) with 50–100% oxygen. Conventional parameters, including heart rate, continuous arterial pressure, central venous pressure, and urine output, are monitored for hemodynamic and fluid management.

Patient Position and Port Placement

The patient is placed in the contralateral decubitus position. Ports are placed according to surgeons' preference. Uniportal or multiportal pulmonary sleeve resections have been demonstrated by many researchers [6–8]. A uniportal access window is usually placed at the fourth or fifth intercostal space along the anterior axillary line. I usually use a triple-port approach: a cam-

K. Kim et al. (eds.), *Techniques in Minimally Invasive Thoracic Surgery*,
https://doi.org/10.1007/978-981-19-2472-9_5

era port at the seventh intercostal space along the mid-axillary line, a posterior port at the sixth intercostal space along the posterior axillary line, and an access window, approximately 5 cm long, at the fifth intercostal space along the anterior axillary line.

Surgical Procedures

The pulmonary artery or vein is isolated and divided in accordance with techniques standard for VATS lobectomy. All pulmonary arterial and venous branches of the target lobe are divided before transection of the bronchus. Regional and mediastinal lymph nodes are completely dissected according to oncologic principles. The bronchus is isolated until surgical margins are sufficient. The bronchial tree around target bronchus is carefully dissected until normal tissue is encountered. The proximal and distal bronchial margin should be guaranteed. Tissue from circumferential bronchial margins are obtained with a knife and scissors and evaluated in frozen biopsy before the bronchial anastomosis. For example, for right upper lobe sleeve lobectomy, the right main and intermediate bronchi should be cancer free. To evaluate for the possibility of end-to-end anastomosis, the bronchial ends are carefully evaluated for size mismatch, gaps between the bronchial stumps, and other obstacles. A hilar or distal dissection can be made to release tension on the anastomosis site. Sometimes, a pericardial incision over the pulmonary vein can be added to release tension. Simple trimming or edging of the stumps can be attempted to overcome caliber disparity. Bronchial flaps from the distal bronchial end and reefing of the membranous portion of the bronchus to adjust caliber mismatch have also been reported [9, 10].

Either absorbable or nonabsorbable suture material can be used for bronchial end-to-end anastomosis. Either running or interrupted sutures can be placed; interrupted sutures are reliable and can enable a good healing process. Recent reports have suggested that continuous sutures can enable comparable outcomes [11–13]. The time to perform anastomosis is short with running sutures, but anastomosis dehiscence can result from bronchial tears at the suture site. I usually use 4-0 absorbable material such as absorbable polyglactin 10 (Vicryl®; Ethicon, Inc., Somerville, NJ, USA), braided absorbable suture (Polysorb™; Medtronic, Dublin, Ireland), or polydioxanone (PDS® II; Ethicon, Inc.) for interrupted sutures. Usually, anastomosis suturing starts at the cartilaginous–membranous junction, which is the site deepest from the surgeon's perspective. The initial two stitches on the cartilage side can afford firm approximation of both bronchial ends. While the sutures are placed with a knot pusher, the distal bronchial end is tucked into the proximal bronchial end to complete telescope anastomosis. Interrupt sutures are placed from the cartilaginous portion to the membranous portion. Usually, 8–10 interrupted sutures are sufficient. After the last suture is tied, air leakage should be tested with normal saline. Additional sutures can be placed at points of air leakage. The anastomosis can be covered with pericardial fat, pericardium, or intercostal muscle.

5.3 Video Clips

Right Middle Lobe Sleeve Lobectomy

After exploration of right thoracic cavity, interlobar lymph nodes are dissected (Fig. 5.1a). The right middle pulmonary artery branches are dissected and isolated from the interlobar pulmonary artery. All medial and lateral pulmonary arterial branches are encircled and divided with one endo-stapler (Fig. 5.1b). The minor fissure is developed with an endo-stapler (Fig. 5.1c). The right middle lobar bronchus is isolated and cut at its origin. In this case, the endobronchial lesion was attached to the bronchial margin that I decided to proceed with sleeve lobectomy. The pulmonary venous branches in the right middle lobe are isolated and divided with an endo-stapler (Fig. 5.1d). Sleeve transection of the bronchus intermedius is performed. The bronchus intermedius is isolated and divided below the origin of

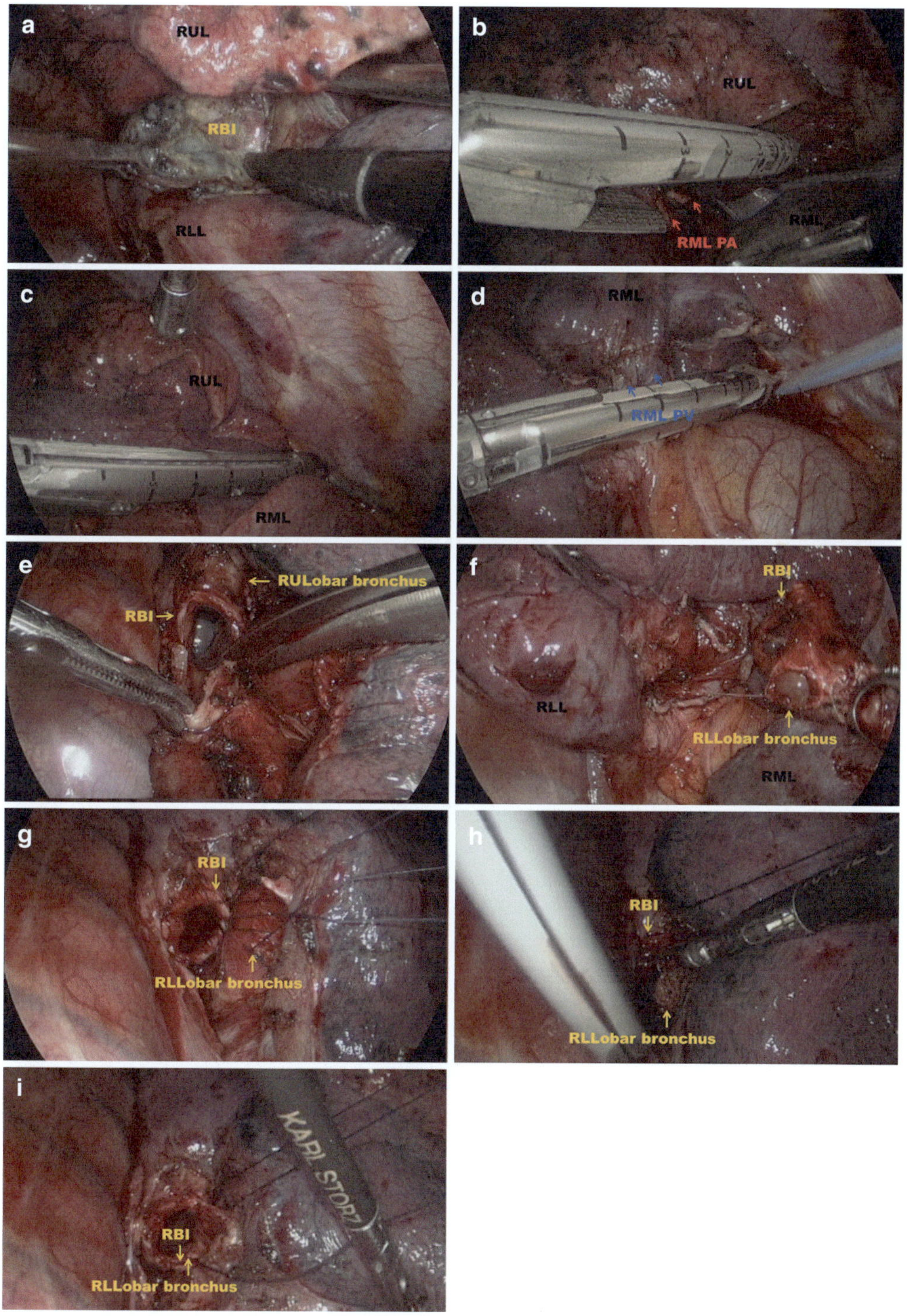

Fig. 5.1 Right middle sleeve lobectomy, performed as video-assisted thoracoscopic surgery. (**a**) Dissection of interlobar lymph nodes. (**b**) Division of pulmonary artery branches of the right middle lobe. (**c**) Division of the minor fissure. (**d**) Division of branches of the pulmonary vein in the right middle lobe. (**e**) Transection of the bronchus intermedius. (**f**) Retrieval of the right middle lobe with the bronchus intermedius. (**g**) Placement of interrupted 4-0 absorbable sutures on cartilaginous portions of the bronchus intermedius and right lower lobar bronchus. (**h**) Tying of the sutures with an endoscopic knot pusher while the right lower lobar bronchus is tucked into the bronchus intermedius. (**i**) Creation of the telescope anastomosis

the right upper lobar bronchus (Fig. 5.1e). The right lower lobar bronchus is then divided at its origin. The right middle lobe is retrieved with the transected bronchus intermedius (Fig. 5.1f) and sent for frozen biopsy of bronchial margins. While the biopsy results are awaited, the mediastinal lymph nodes are dissected. After clear bronchial resection margins are confirmed by biopsy, bronchial reconstruction is performed. To begin the bronchial end-to-end anastomosis, sutures are placed on the cartilaginous–membranous junction. I place two rows of 4-0 Polysorb® interrupted sutures on the bronchial cartilage (Fig. 5.1g). While the sutures are knotted with an endoscopic knot pusher, the right lower lobar bronchus is tucked into the bronchus intermedius (Fig. 5.1h) to accomplish a telescope anastomosis (Fig. 5.1i). Each knot is tied just after the next suture to prevent threads from tangling. Stitch intervals are adjusted to even the distribution of tension according to the calibers of each bronchial end. After completion of bronchial reconstruction, the lack of air leaks in the anastomosis is confirmed by an underwater test.

Left Lower Lobe Sleeve Lobectomy

VATS for left lower lobar sleeve lobectomy is identical to VATS for left lower lobectomy, except for bronchial management. After exploration of the thoracic cavity, the minor fissure is dissected and divided with endo-staplers. The branches of the pulmonary artery in the left lower lobe are isolated and divided with an endo-stapler (Fig. 5.2a), as is the left inferior pulmonary vein (Fig. 5.2b). The left lower lobar bronchus is isolated and transected at its orifice (Fig. 5.2c). In this case, the endobronchial lesion was involved to the bronchial margin that I decided to proceed with sleeve lobectomy. Sleeve transection of the bronchus is performed. The distal left main bronchus is divided with a scalpel just before the origin of the left upper lobar bronchus (Fig. 5.2d). The left upper lobar bronchus is trimmed. The proximal and distal bronchia margins are sent for frozen biopsy to confirm that the margins were clear. During the biopsy, the mediastinal lymph nodes are dissected. After clear bronchial resection margins are confirmed, bronchial reconstruction is performed. To begin bronchial end-to-end anastomosis, sutures are placed on the cartilaginous–membranous junction. Two rows of 4-0 Polysorb® interrupted sutures were placed on the bronchial cartilage (Fig. 5.2e). While a knot is made with an endoscopic knot pusher, the left upper lobar bronchus is tucked into the left main bronchus. Interrupted sutures are then placed in the membranous portion (Fig. 5.2f) in concentric circles, extending to the anterior wall (Fig. 5.2g). Stitch intervals are adjusted according to the calibers of each bronchial end. After bronchial reconstruction is completed, the lack of air leaks in the anastomosis is confirmed by an underwater test.

Techniques for sleeve lobectomy in other lobes are described in several other reports [13, 14].

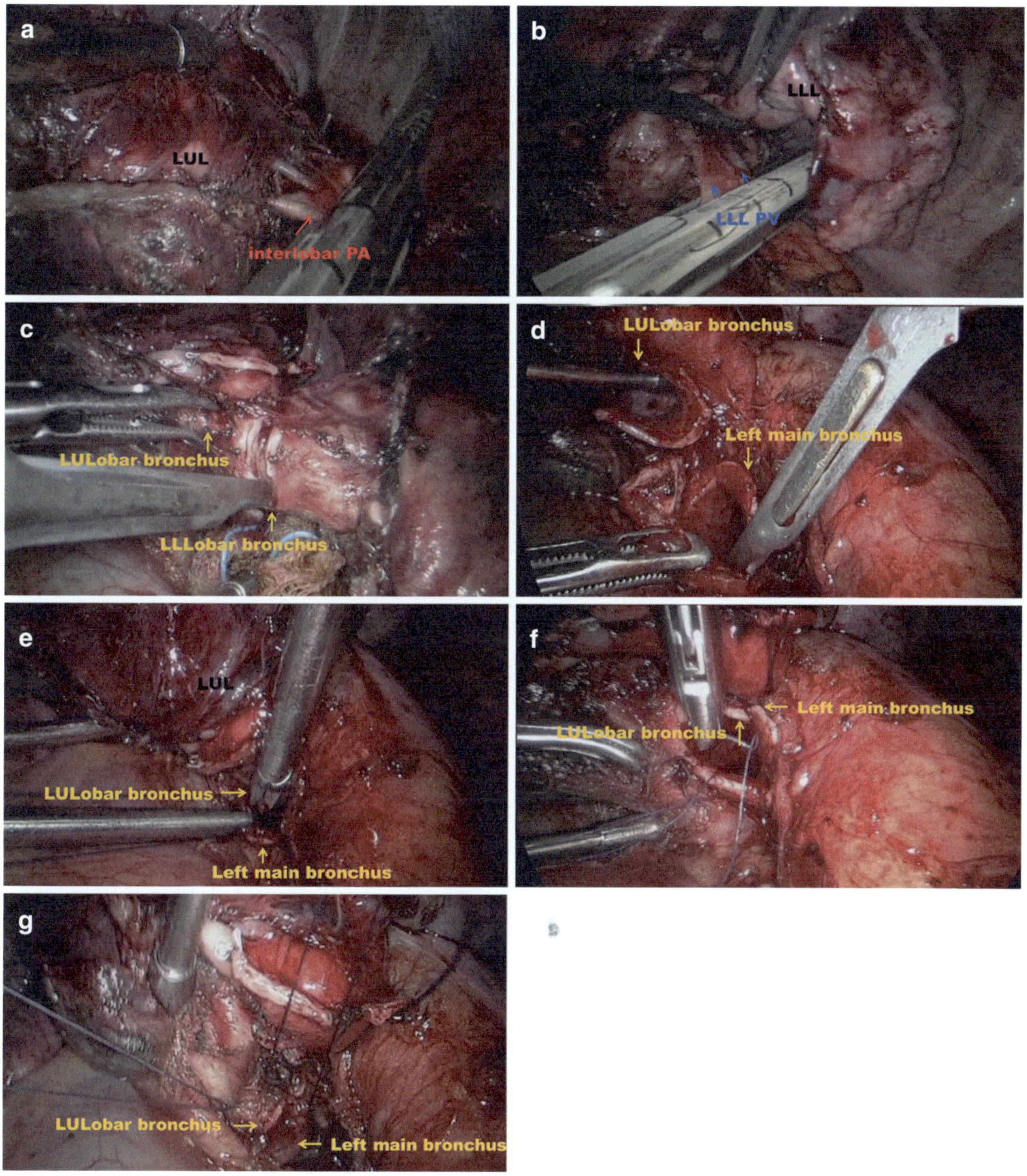

Fig. 5.2 Left lower lobe sleeve lobectomy, performed as video-assisted thoracoscopic surgery. (**a**) Division of branches of the pulmonary artery in the left lower lobe. (**b**) Division of the left inferior pulmonary vein. (**c**) Transection of the left lower lobar bronchus at its orifice. (**d**) Transection of the distal left main bronchus. (**e**) Placement of interrupted sutures on cartilaginous portions of the left main bronchus and the left upper lobar bronchus. (**f**) Placement of interrupted sutures on the membranous portion. (**g**) Completion of bronchial end-to-end anastomosis at anterior wall of bronchus. *RUL* right upper lobe, *RML* right middle lobe, *RLL* right lower lobe, *LUL* left upper lobe, *LLL* left lower lobe, *RBI* right bronchus intermedius, *PA* pulmonary artery, *PV* pulmonary vein

5.4 Conclusion

Pulmonary sleeve lobectomy is a complex procedure that requires technical skills. VATS bronchial sleeve lobectomy is technically challenging; however, much experience has been accumulated. Various techniques to overcome difficulties during VATS sleeve lobectomy have been reported. Surgical principles of sleeve lobectomy in thoracotomy should be applied equally in VATS procedures.

Acknowledgements None.

Conflict of Interest None.

Funding None.

References

1. Thomas CP. Conservative resection of the bronchial tree. J R Coll Surg Edinb. 1956;1(3):169–86.
2. Thomas CP. Conservative and extensive resection for carcinoma of the lung. Ann R Coll Surg Engl. 1959;24(6):345–65.
3. Yoshino I, Yokoyama H, Yano T, et al. Comparison of the surgical results of lobectomy with bronchoplasty and pneumonectomy for lung cancer. J Surg Oncol. 1997;64(1):32–5.
4. Okada M, Yamagishi H, Satake S, et al. Survival related to lymph node involvement in lung cancer after sleeve lobectomy compared with pneumonectomy. J Thorac Cardiovasc Surg. 2000;119(4 Pt 1):814–9.
5. He J, Shao W, Cao C, et al. Long-term outcome of hybrid surgical approach of video-assisted thoracic minithoracotomy sleeve lobectomy for non-small cell lung cancer. Surg Endosc. 2011;25:2509–15.
6. Santambrogio L, Cioffi U, De Simone M, Rosso L, Ferrero S, Giunta A. Video-assisted sleeve lobectomy for mucoepidermoid carcinoma of the left lower lobar bronchus: a case report. Chest. 2002;121(2):635–6. https://doi.org/10.1378/chest.121.2.635.
7. Gonzalez-rivas D, Fernandez R, Fieira E. Uniportal video-assisted thoracoscopic bronchial sleeve lobectomy: first report. J Thorac Cardiovasc Surg. 2013;145(6):1676–7.
8. Koryllos A, Stoelben E. Uniportal video-assisted thoracoscopic surgery (VATS) sleeve resections for non-small cell lung cancer patients: an observational prospective study and technique analysis. J Vis Surg. 2018;4:16.
9. Ohata K, Zhang J, Ito S, Yoshimura T, Matsubara Y, Terada Y. Right lower lobe sleeve resection: bronchial flap to correct caliber disparity. Ann Thorac Surg. 2013;95(3):1107–8. https://doi.org/10.1016/j.athoracsur.2012.09.083.
10. Toyooka S, Soh J, Oto T, Miyoshi S. Bronchoplasty to adjust mismatches in the proximal and distal bronchial stumps during bronchial sleeve resection of the left lower lobe and lingular division. Eur J Cardiothorac Surg. 2013;43(1):182–3. https://doi.org/10.1093/ejcts/ezs379.
11. Kutlu CA, Goldstraw P. Tracheobronchial sleeve resection with the use of a continuous anastomosis: results of one hundred consecutive cases. J Thorac Cardiovasc Surg. 1999;117:1112–7.
12. Igai H, Yokomise H. Bronchoplasty with continuous sutures for non-small-cell lung cancer. Gen Thorac Cardiovasc Surg. 2012;60:249–51.
13. Yang R, Shao F, Cao H, Liu Z. Bronchial anastomosis using complete continuous suture in video-assisted thoracic surgery sleeve lobectomy. J Thorac Dis. 2013;5:S321–2.
14. Huang J, Li S, Hao Z, et al. Complete video-assisted thoracoscopic surgery (VATS) bronchial sleeve lobectomy. J Thorac Dis. 2016;8(3):553–74. https://doi.org/10.21037/jtd.2016.01.63.

Video-Assisted Thoracic Surgery for Pneumonectomy

6

Seokjin Haam

Abstract

Video-assisted thoracic surgery (VATS) for lobectomy or segmentectomy is considered as a good alternative to thoracotomy because of its usefulness and safety; reducing postoperative pain, lowering morbidity, and shortening hospital stay. However, despite these advantages of VATS, it has been difficult to perform VATS pneumonectomy due to the high morbidity and mortality rate of pneumonectomy. Recently, as VATS technique has been developed and usefulness of VATS pneumonectomy has been continuously reported, VATS pneumonectomy is gradually increasing in large volume centers. This article describes VATS pneumonectomy with a focus on the surgical technique.

Keywords

Video-assisted thoracic surgery
Pneumonectomy · Surgical technique
Intraoperative management

S. Haam (✉)
Department of Thoracic and Cardiovascular Surgery, Ajou University Hospital, Ajou University School of Medicine, Suwon, Republic of Korea
e-mail: haamsj@aumc.ac.kr

6.1 Introduction

Over the last two decades, the video-assisted thoracic surgery (VATS) technique has become the main treatment option for peripheral small lung nodules as well as major lung resection, including lobectomy. However, because complications observed after pneumonectomy were thought to be caused by the large amount of lung tissue resected rather than by the differences in the surgical method, VATS pneumonectomy was not actively performed compared to VATS lobectomy. This has contributed to our limited understanding of whether the advantages of VATS in lobectomy are also apparent in pneumonectomy. However, according to recent studies, VATS pneumonectomy is not inferior to open pneumonectomy in oncologic aspects and leads to superior results in postoperative pain and recovery [1]. In locally advanced lung cancer where pneumonectomy is the main treatment option, adjuvant therapy must be started as early as possible after operation; thus, postoperative pain management and rapid recovery are important [2]. For these reasons, VATS pneumonectomy has greater advantages over open pneumonectomy [3].

K. Kim et al. (eds.), *Techniques in Minimally Invasive Thoracic Surgery*,
https://doi.org/10.1007/978-981-19-2472-9_6

6.2 Indications for VATS Pneumonectomy

Similar to open pneumonectomy, the main indication for VATS pneumonectomy is locally advanced lung cancer that cannot be completely resected by lobectomy, bilobectomy, or sleeve lobectomy. Patients must be able to tolerate one-lung ventilation during the surgery and have sufficient lung function for their daily lives after pneumonectomy. VATS pneumonectomy should not be performed when complete resection is impossible, even with pneumonectomy or in patients with positive N3 nodes. Although there are no absolute criteria for the mass size, VATS must be carefully considered for large masses. In addition, VATS pneumonectomy should be carefully considered in patients who underwent preoperative chemotherapy or chemoradiation therapy and resection of the opposite lung.

6.3 Preoperative Evaluation

The preoperative evaluation for VATS pneumonectomy is similar to that for open pneumonectomy: a transthoracic echocardiogram and pulmonary function test. In patients with marginal functions whose condition cannot accurately be evaluated using these routine tests, a supplementary lung perfusion or cardiopulmonary exercise test must be conducted. For a more accurate assessment of the cardiopulmonary function, the pulmonary artery (PA) on the side to be resected may be ballooned during cardiac catheterization to analyze cardiac output, right ventricular function, and systemic arterial blood gas. And, cardiac function can be evaluated by clamping the main PA under the intraoperative transesophageal echocardiogram.

6.4 Anesthesia

VATS pneumonectomy is performed under general anesthesia using one-lung ventilation. General anesthesia is induced through inhalation or intravenous injection of anesthetic agents, after which the patient is intubated with a double lumen endotracheal tube. The double lumen endotracheal tube tip can be placed in either side of the main bronchus depending on the resection side; however, if the tip enters the main bronchus in the resection direction, the tip can also be resected during main bronchus resection. Therefore, the anesthesiologist must inform the surgeon about the direction of the tube tip prior to bronchus resection.

Intraoperative hypoxemia requires special considerations for VATS pneumonectomy. In open pneumonectomy, continuous positive airway pressure can be applied to the non-ventilated lung to improve hypoxia. However, during VATS pneumonectomy, the same procedure cannot be performed as it can limit the visual field and movement of the instruments. Therefore, hypoxemia during VATS pneumonectomy can be corrected by applying positive end expiatory pressure or conducting intermittent two-lung ventilation after discussing with the surgeon.

In order to minimize injury of the opposite (non-resected) lung after pneumonectomy, airway pressure must be maintained at a low level and the inhaled oxygen concentration must be minimized during the surgery. In addition, intravenous fluids must not be infused in large quantities [4].

6.5 Surgical Technique

General Concept

Right VATS pneumonectomy has a higher risk of postoperative respiratory failure and bronchopleural fistula (BPF) than left VATS pneumonectomy; however, right VATS pneumonectomy is technically easier than left side because the pulmonary vasculature and carina are well-exposed. As the extracted specimen is often larger in VATS pneumonectomy than in lobectomy, specimens may not be obtained using the usual VATS incision. In this case, it may be necessary to extend the incision for extraction.

During pneumonectomy, both inferior and superior pulmonary veins (PV) must be sufficiently isolated before the division of one of these veins. This can isolate and divide the main PA without delay after the division of the two PV. This technique reduces the time required to isolate and divide the PA, thereby preventing vascular congestion.

In completion pneumonectomy or cases of deep mass invasion toward the center, vessels may need to be divided inside the pericardium. In bronchus division, as in open pneumonectomy, dissection must be done until the carinal level to ensure that the bronchus stump is as short as possible.

Patient Positioning

The position of the patients is the same as in VATS lobectomy. The patients need to be in a full lateral decubitus position, and the operation bed is flexed. This widens the intercostal space (ICS) and improves access and control of thoracoscopic devices.

Incision

The number and location of incisions differ for each surgeon. Here, we will introduce a general three-port technique. First, a trocar is inserted to the eighth ICS posterior axillary line and the sixth ICS anterior axillary line, respectively. The thoracoscope and thoracoscopic devices are inserted through these trocars to observe the inside of the thoracic cavity. After confirming the location and invasion extent of the tumor to assess indications for VATS pneumonectomy, a 4-cm-long working window is created at the fifth ICS. If surgery is contraindicated due to pleural metastasis, the surgery needs to be terminated. If VATS cannot be performed, conversion to thoracotomy is necessary.

Division of Pulmonary Veins

There is a controversy over whether the PV or artery must be divided first. If the PV is divided first, pulmonary congestion may occur. On the other hand, if the PA is divided first, the cancer cells may metastasize through the bloodstream during surgery [5]. Technically, the division of the PV prior to that of the PA leads to an easier and safer exposure and division of the PA.

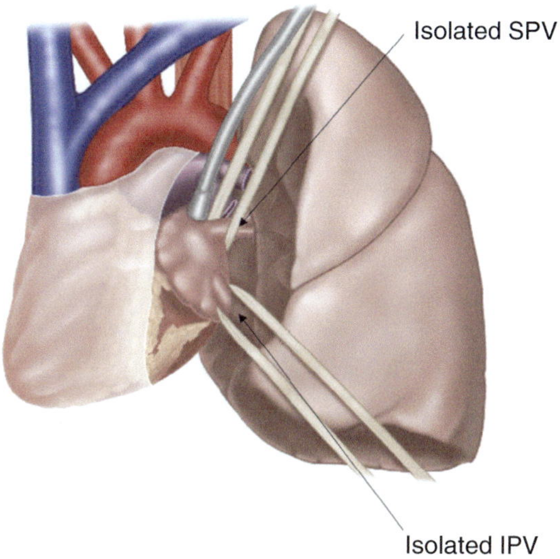

Fig. 6.1 The inferior pulmonary ligament is dissected up to the bottom of the inferior pulmonary vein (IPV). IPV is encircled with vessel loop or umbilical tape. After division of IPV, the lower boundary of the superior pulmonary vein is well-exposed. *SPV* superior pulmonary vein

To divide the PV, the inferior pulmonary ligament must be dissected up to the bottom of the inferior PV (IPV). Once the IPV is exposed, vessel loops or umbilical tape can be used to encircle the IPV, which can then be divided using a stapler. When the IPV is divided, the lower boundary of the superior PV (SPV) is well-exposed (Fig. 6.1). As the SPV is in very close proximity with the anterior part of the PA, caution is required to avoid injury of the PA during encircling. The SPV can be divided using a stapler in the same way as the IPV.

Division of Pulmonary Artery

After lifting the lung upward and exposing the lower parts of the PA and bronchus, the space between the PA and bronchus can be dissected. The lung can be retracted downward to expose

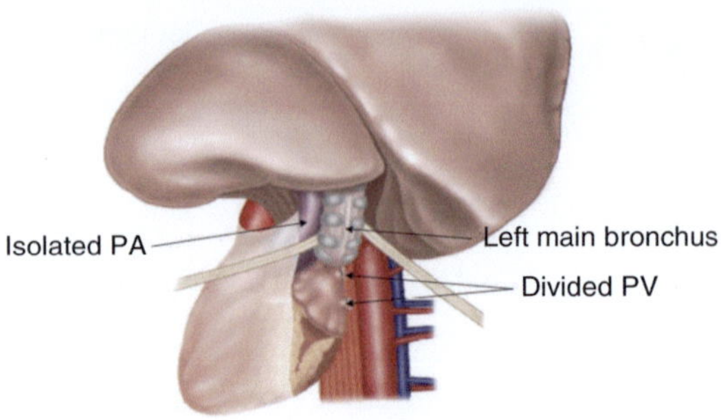

Fig. 6.2 Dissecting tissues around the upper part of the pulmonary artery (PA), and the lung is retracted superiorly. After creating a space between the PA and main bronchus, vessel loop is placed in this space. *PV* pulmonary vein

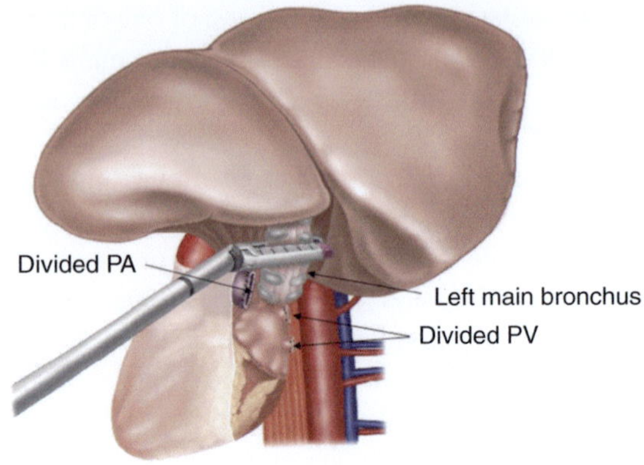

Fig. 6.3 Because long bronchus stump can cause bronchopleural fistula, it is essential to keep the bronchus stump as short as possible. When bronchus is divided before pulmonary artery (PA) division, the PA may rotate or be pulled, leading to injuries. PA division is generally conducted before bronchus division. *PV* pulmonary vein

the subaortic area. After dissecting tissues around the upper part of the PA, the PA is encircled. After encircling the vessel loop or umbilical tape, enough space must be secured for the stapler to pass through (Fig. 6.2). If the tissues around the PA are not dissected properly, the staplers may cause vessel injuries. In rare cases, the stapler may distort the main PA or contralateral PA. Therefore, the PA should not be divided immediately after closure, and changes in hemodynamics must be observed for a sufficient time before PA division. If the mass is located too close to the origin of the PA, it may be difficult to place the stapler. In such cases, intrapericardial division can be considered and it is safe to proceed with conversion to thoracotomy.

Division of Bronchus

As described earlier, it is essential to keep the bronchus stump as short as possible. In the left lung, the bronchus in the subaortic area must be sufficiently dissected to leave a short bronchus stump. Dissection of the subcarinal node after bronchus division makes it technically challenging to expose the subcarinal area. Therefore, it is better to perform node dissection before bronchus division. During dissection of the subcarinal node, a clip or scissors are recommended over energy devices, which may cause devascularization. When bronchus is divided before PA division, the PA may rotate or be pulled, leading to injuries. Therefore, in general, PA division is conducted before bronchus division (Fig. 6.3). However, if the mass is located in front of the PA, limiting hilar dissection, bronchus division can be performed first. Excessive dissection of the tissue at the bronchus resection margin impairs blood circulation, which increases the risk of BPF. In VATS pneumonectomy, extraction of the lung specimen is challenging. Extracting the specimen through a narrow working window may damage the bag, which can cause the dissemination of cancer cells. In this case, the intercostal muscle must be divided sufficiently such that the specimen can be extracted safely to the subcutaneous space. Cancers that require VATS pneumonectomy may be located close to the bronchus resection margin. Thus, frozen sections of the bronchus margin need to be requested for examination by the pathologist. If cancer cells are present in the margin, additional resection of the bronchus stump may be necessary.

Coverage of Drainage after Bronchus Stump

Once the lung specimens are extracted, the thoracic cavity is irrigated with warm saline. Some surgeons may also mix antibiotics with the irrigation fluid. During irrigation, air leakage in the bronchus must be checked. If an air leakage is observed, the bronchus can be sutured or stapled again. Subsequently, some surgeons may cover the bronchus stump with surrounding tissues rich in blood vessels. Commonly used tissues are pericardial fat pads, pleura, and intercostal muscles. Since right pneumonectomy and neoadjuvant treatment induce a high risk of BFF, it is safer to cover the stump.

Drainage After VATS Pneumonectomy

Although drainage after pneumonectomy can be done in various ways, the necessity of drainage is also debated. In general, a chest tube connected to a three-bottle system is commonly used. Inserting drains can help control mediastinum positioning immediately after surgery, and it is useful to identify the characteristics of the drained content, such as blood and chyle. The chest tube is not maintained for a long time unless complications are observed in the immediate postoperative period.

6.6 Postoperative Management

Pleural Space After Pneumonectomy

After VATS pneumonectomy, fluids accumulate in the empty thoracic cavity. On chest radiographs, approximately 70% of the thoracic cavity is commonly filled with fluid on the third postoperative day, and 2–3 months are required for the thoracic cavity to be completely filled with fluid [6]. Rapid postoperative fluid accumulation indicates possible bleeding and chylothorax. If the mediastinum is severely deviated to the opposite side of the operation, the subcutaneous emphysema is suddenly aggravated or fluid does not fill above the carinal level, BPF should be suspected.

Fluid Management

An excessive fluid supply during or after surgery increases the possibility of pulmonary edema in the remaining lung, which is associated with postoperative mortality. As described above, severe fluid restriction is also dangerous as the thoracic cavity is filled with fluid within a short period of time. The urine output and renal function must be closely monitored to supply appropriate amounts of fluid.

6.7 Conclusion

VATS pneumonectomy is often conducted for patients with locally advanced lung cancer with central lesions. The surgical technique is complex, and the risk of postoperative complications limits the use of VATS pneumonectomy compared to VATS lobectomy. However, the gradual development of the VATS technique and experience would help to replace open pneumonectomy for the treatment of lung cancer in the near future.

Conflict of Interest None.

References

1. Nwogu CE, Yendamuri S, Demmy TL. Does thoracoscopic pneumonectomy for lung cancer affect survival? Ann Thorac Surg. 2010;89:S2102–6.
2. Petersen RP, Pham D, Burfeind WR, et al. Thoracoscopic lobectomy facilitates the delivery of chemotherapy after resection for lung cancer. Ann Thorac Surg. 2007;83:1245–50.
3. Yang CJ, Yendamuri S, Mayne NR, et al. The role of thoracoscopic pneumonectomy in the management of non-small cell lung cancer: a multicenter study. J Thorac Cardiovasc Surg. 2019;158:252–64.
4. Hackett S, Jones R, Kapila R. Anaesthesia for pneumonectomy. BJA Educ. 2019;19:297–304.
5. Song PP, Zhang W, Zhang B, Liu Q, Du J. Effects of different sequences of pulmonary artery and vein ligations during pulmonary lobectomy on blood micrometastasis of non-small cell lung cancer. Oncol Lett. 2013;5:463–8.
6. Munden RF, O'Sullivan PJ, Liu P, Vaporciyan AA. Radiographic evaluation of the pleural fluid accumulation rate after pneumonectomy. Clin Imaging. 2015;39:247–50.

7 Video-Assisted Thoracic Surgery Mediastinal Lymph Node Dissection in Lung Cancer Surgery

Kwhanmien Kim

Abstract

Mediastinal lymph node dissection is an important part of lung cancer surgery that provides accurate nodal staging and may improve survival outcomes. The minimally invasive approach, such as video-assisted thoracic surgery (VATS) lobectomy for patients with non-small cell lung cancer, has become a standard operation worldwide. VATS mediastinal lymph node dissection should be thorough and accurate to ensure the completeness of lung cancer surgery. Herein, the author describes techniques for VATS mediastinal lymph node dissection.

Keywords

Lung neoplasms · Video-assisted thoracic surgery · Lymph node dissection

7.1 Introduction

Lymph node dissection, including the hilar and mediastinal lymph nodes, is an important procedure in non-small cell lung cancer surgery. Mediastinal lymph node dissection (MLND) is crucial for achieving complete surgery. Although whether MLND can increase survival has yet to be conclusively established, it can provide accurate pathological staging and better local control [1, 2]. Complete lymph node dissection can be defined as the removal of all lymph nodes and fat tissues from each nodal station. The video-assisted thoracic surgery (VATS) lymph node dissection technique is almost the same as that of open thoracotomy, but it can vary according to the position of the thoracoscope, the presence of a working window, the surgical instruments used, and the adequacy of the surgical view provided by the thoracoscope. VATS MLND can now be safely performed and enables more lymph nodes to be harvested [3–9]. However, the extent of lymphadenectomy and the requirement of nodal stations for removal according to the lung cancer location have yet to be fully elucidated [10, 11].

7.2 Port Placement

There are many different port placement techniques for VATS lung cancer surgery according to the surgeon's preference. Before making VATS ports, it is important to consider a few points: an ergonomically good position to handle the instruments, ease of conversion to open thoracotomy in an emergency, a cosmetically favorable location, and the need to minimize postoperative pain. The author's standard VATS incisions include two

K. Kim (✉)
Department of Thoracic and Cardiovascular Surgery, Seoul National University Bundang Hospital, Seoul National University College of Medicine, Seonganam, Gyeonggi-Do, Republic of Korea
e-mail: kmkim0070@snubh.org

K. Kim et al. (eds.), *Techniques in Minimally Invasive Thoracic Surgery*,
https://doi.org/10.1007/978-981-19-2472-9_7

ports and one utility incision (working window) [12]. The first port for the initial thoracoscopic exploration is placed at the seventh or eighth intercostal space (ICS) in the mid-axillary line. A working window of about 4 cm in length is placed at the fourth or fifth ICS in the mid-clavicular line. Specially-designed wound retractors are commercially available to enhance instrument handling and prevent wound contamination. An additional 5- or 10-mm port is made at the fifth or sixth ICS below the scapular tip (Fig. 7.1). This port configuration guarantees safe and prompt conversion to open thoracotomy in emergent situations by connecting the working window and the posterior port. Simply by changing the thoracoscope port and applying appropriate maneuvers, all lung lobes can be resected and MLND can be achieved by this 3-port configuration without major modifications. However, the decisions of where to stand, where to introduce the thoracoscope, and whether to change the thoracoscope port or to use a fixed port all depend solely on the surgeon's preference. The most important consideration is to avoid competing with the assistant's instruments (the "no hand cross-over" technique). The author recommends always standing at the right side of the operating table because it allows smooth right-hand maneuvers. When performing left-side VATS lobectomy, a 10-mm port for the thoracoscope is placed in the fifth or sixth ICS along the anterior scapular line, which can provide better fissure development and subcarinal exposure (Fig. 7.2).

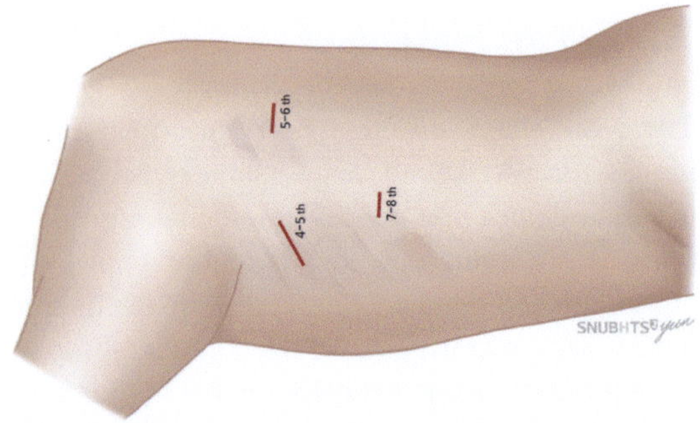

Fig. 7.1 3-Port placement sites on the left side

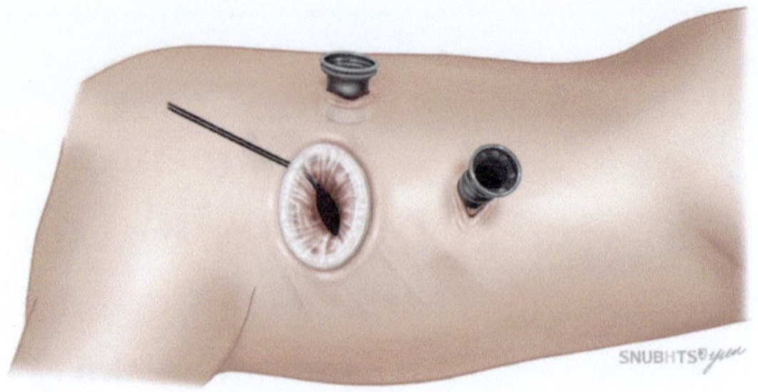
Fig. 7.2 Left-side 3-port placement with a 10-mm trocar in the fifth or sixth intercostal space along the anterior scapular line. If the thoracoscope is introduced through this back port, it can provide better fissure development and subcarinal exposure

7.3 Techniques of VATS Mediastinal Lymph Node Dissection

Right Side

Stations 2R, 3, and 4R

The mediastinal pleura is opened from the junction of the azygos vein and the superior vena cava (SVC). From below the azygos vein to the right brachiocephalic artery, between the trachea and the SVC, a longitudinal incision is made on the parietal pleura. It is easy to dissect all the mediastinal fat tissue, including the lymph nodes, from below the azygos vein to the level of the innominate artery in an upward direction. With elevation of the azygos vein and pushing down the right main pulmonary artery trunk, the mediastinal fat pad between the right main bronchus and anterior carinal area is dissected first, and then the dissection moves on to the pericardium around the aortic arch. The azygos vein is retracted caudally and the SVC is retracted anteriorly with an endoscopic retractor and peanut; the mediastinal fat pad is dissected from the trachea and the SVC and from the caudal border of the innominate artery (Fig. 7.3a, b). All mediastinal fat tissues, including the lymph nodes are removed en bloc. Small veins draining from the mediastinal fat tissues directly into the SVC are ligated with hemoclips or divided with an ultrasonic device. At the

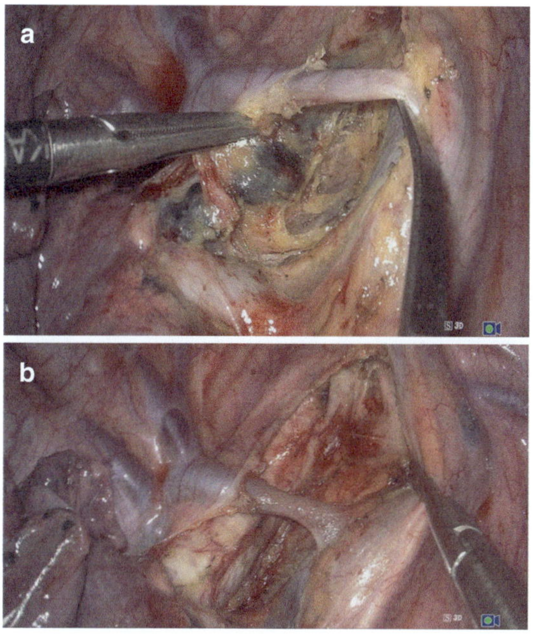

Fig. 7.3 (**a**) Right upper mediastinal dissection starts from below the azygos vein, moving upward. (**b**) After complete node dissection, the mediastinal borders (the trachea, the pericardium, the innominate artery, and the superior vena cava) can be seen

apex, the right recurrent laryngeal nerve can be damaged by thermal injury. Because there are many small lymphatic channels in this area, those should be ligated or treated safely to avoid post-operative chylothorax. The author prefers to use an ultrasonic device, because it is easy to dissect mediastinal fat tissues with less bleeding and it may help to prevent postoperative lymphatic leakage.

Station 7 (Right Side)

After tilting the operating table leftward and retracting the right lung anteriorly, the right subcarinal area is exposed easily. The parietal pleural is then opened, avoiding injury to the vagus nerve and its pulmonary branches. Although the small pulmonary vagal branches running into the bronchus are usually divided, it is better to save those branches to reduce pulmonary complications such as dry cough after operation. The subcarinal fat pad is dissected en bloc, starting inferiorly and moving upward to the carina with electrocautery or ultrasonic devices. Dissection starts from the inferior border of the bronchus intermedius and the inferior pulmonary vein, and then it moves upward. Then, subcarinal lymph nodes are dissected from the esophagus and the left and right main bronchi. The anterior subcarinal space can be reached by an anterior approach if clear dissection is difficult from behind (Fig. 7.4a, b).

Left Side

Stations 5 and 6

The mediastinal pleura is opened between the phrenic and the vagus nerves at the level of the aortopulmonary window. The incision is extended along the vagus nerve in a cephalad direction and horizontally above the left main pulmonary artery. Attention should be paid to avoid the phrenic nerve and left recurrent laryngeal nerve injuries. The level 6 lymph nodes are located in the area medial to the ligamentum arteriosum and the level 5 lymph nodes are between the lower border of the aortic arch and the upper rim of the left main pulmonary artery. The aortopulmonary fat pad containing the level 5 and 6 lymph nodes is removed en bloc (Fig. 7.5).

Station 4L

The left paratracheal lymph nodes are located between the upper margin of the aortic arch and the upper rim of the left main pulmonary artery. After pushing down the left main pulmonary artery with a peanut and retracting the aortic arch upward with an endoscopic retractor, the 4L lymph nodes are dissected along the left main bronchus to the trachea. The 4L lymph nodes are close to the left recurrent laryngeal nerve. To avoid left vocal cord palsy, the left recurrent laryngeal nerve and the proximal vagus nerve must be carefully preserved (Fig. 7.6).

Station 7 (Left Side)

It is a little more difficult to expose the left sub-carinal space because of the longer left main bronchus, the descending aorta, and the spine. A right-sided double-lumen endotracheal intubation is necessary to facilitate the elevation of the

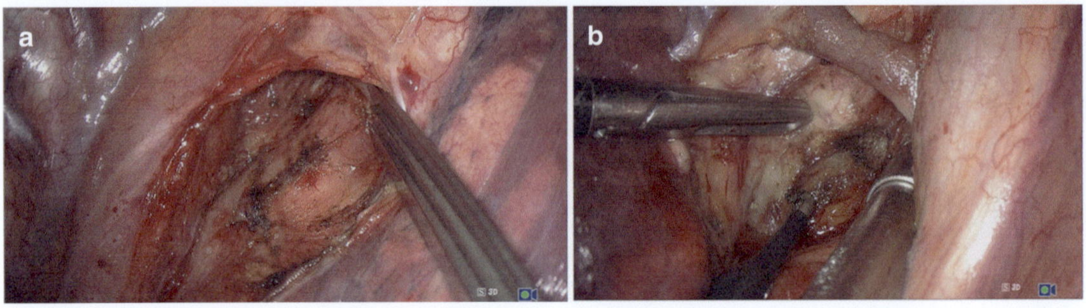

Fig. 7.4 (**a**) Right-side subcarinal lymph node dissection is performed while saving the vagus nerve pulmonary branches through the posterior approach. (**b**) The anterior subcarinal space can be reached through the anterior approach if clear dissection is difficult from behind

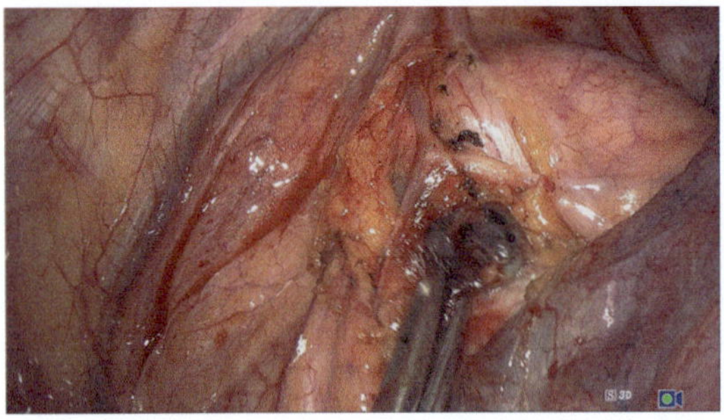

Fig. 7.5 Subaortic and paraaortic lymph nodes are dissected with care taken for the phrenic and left recurrent laryngeal nerves

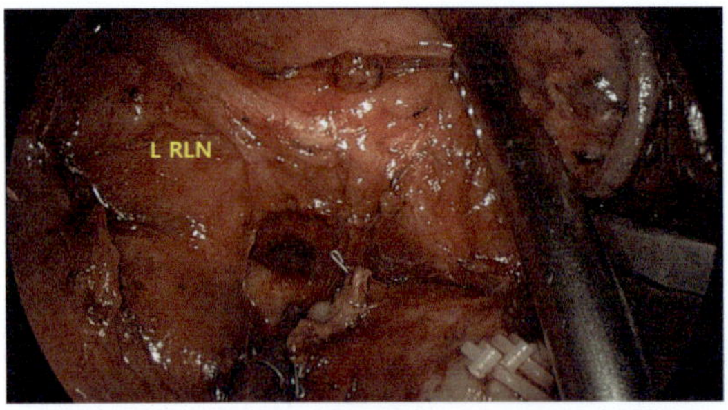

Fig. 7.6 The left recurrent laryngeal nerve (L RLN) is safely preserved after dissection of subaortic and left lower paratracheal lymph nodes

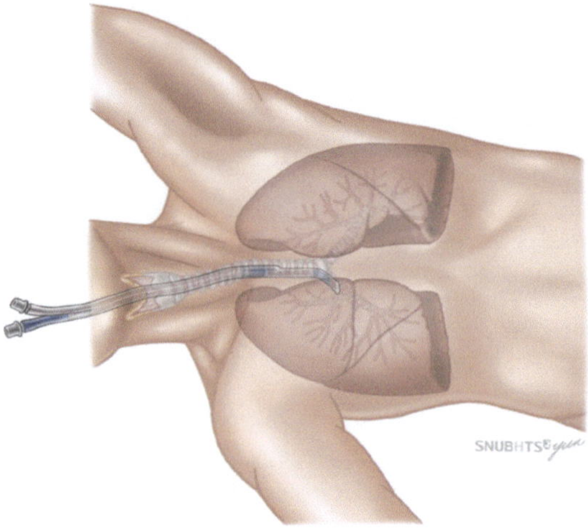

Fig. 7.7 Right-side double-lumen intubation can facilitate subcarinal lymph node dissection during left-side video-assisted thoracic surgery for lung cancer

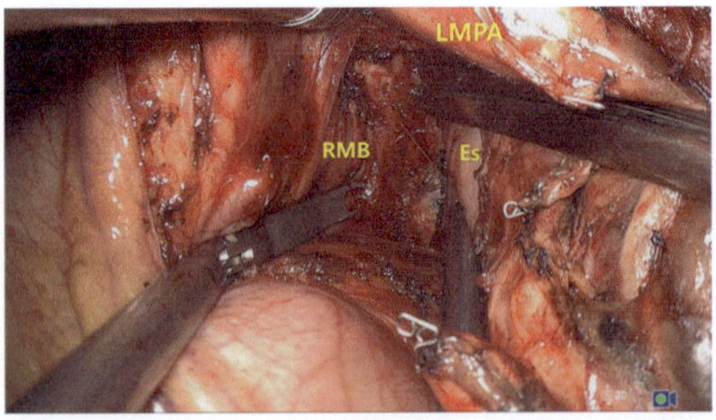

Fig. 7.8 The left subcarinal space can be approached anteriorly while elevating the left main bronchus and the left main pulmonary artery and pushing down the superior pulmonary vein stump, especially after left upper lobectomy. *RMB* right main bronchus, *LMPA* left main pulmonary artery, *Es* esophagus

left main bronchus during the left subcarinal lymph node dissection (Fig. 7.7). The left subcarinal space can be approached anteriorly with the lung retracted posteriorly and elevating the left main bronchus and the left main pulmonary artery, especially after left upper lobectomy (Fig. 7.8). When the left lower lobectomy is performed, the left subcarinal space is approached posteriorly. The mediastinal pleura is opened anterior to and along the descending aorta. The small branches of the vagus nerve supplying the lung are divided. To expose the left subcarinal space, the left main bronchus is retracted anteriorly with an endoscopic fan retractor or endoscopic peanut, and the descending aorta and the esophagus are retracted posteriorly with an endoscopic esophageal retractor. The subcarinal fat pad is dissected from the left main bronchus to the carina. Lymph node dissection is then carried out from the esophagus and the right main bronchus. The small arterial branches entering the lymph nodes from the anterior border of the trachea at the level of the carina should be treated properly to avoid postoperative bleeding.

Conflict of Interest No potential conflict of interest relevant to this article was reported.

References

1. Keller SM, Adak S, Wagner H, Johnson DH. Mediastinal lymph node dissection improves survival in patients with stages II and IIIa non-small cell lung cancer. Ann Thorac Surg. 2000;70:358–65.
2. Allen MS, Darling GE, Pechet TT, et al. Morbidity and mortality of major pulmonary resections in patients with early-stage lung cancer: initial results of the randomized, prospective ACOSOG Z0030 trial. Ann Thorac Surg. 2006;81:1013–9.
3. Watanabe A, Koyanagi T, Ohsawa H, et al. Systematic node dissection by VATS is not inferior to that through an open thoracotomy: a comparative clinicopathologic retrospective study. Surgery. 2005;138:510–7.
4. Sagawa M, Sato M, Sakurada A, et al. A prospective trial of systematic nodal dissection for lung cancer by video-assisted thoracic surgery: can it be perfect? Ann Thorac Surg. 2002;73:900–4.
5. Palade E, Passlick B, Osei-Agyemang T, Gunter J, Wiesemann S. Video-assisted vs open mediastinal lymphadenectomy for stage I non-small-cell lung cancer: results of a prospective randomized trial. Eur J Cardiothorac Surg. 2013;44:244–9.
6. Lee HS, Jang HJ. Thoracoscopic mediastinal lymph node dissection for lung cancer. Semin Thorac Cardiovasc Surg. 2012;24:131–41.
7. Kim K, Kim HK, Park JS, et al. Video-assisted thoracic surgery lobectomy: single institutional experience with 704 cases. Ann Thorac Surg. 2010;89:S2118–22.
8. Kim HK, Choi YS, Kim J, Shim YM, Kim K. Outcomes of unexpected pathologic N1 and N2 disease after video-assisted thoracic surgery lobectomy for clinical stage I non-small cell lung cancer. J Thorac Cardiovasc Surg. 2010;140:1288–93.
9. Amer K. Thoracoscopic mediastinal lymph node dissection for lung cancer. Semin Thorac Cardiovasc Surg. 2012;24:74–8.
10. Shapiro M, Kadakia S, Lim J, et al. Lobe-specific mediastinal nodal dissection is sufficient during lobectomy by video-assisted thoracic surgery or thoracotomy for early-stage lung cancer. Chest. 2013;144:1615–21.
11. Ishiguro F, Matsuo K, Fukui T, Mori S, Hatooka S, Mitsudomi T. Effect of selective lymph node dissection based on patterns of lobe-specific lymph node metastases on patient outcome in patients with resectable non-small cell lung cancer: a large-scale retrospective cohort study applying a propensity score. J Thorac Cardiovasc Surg. 2010;139:1001–6.
12. Kim K. VATS mediastinal lymph node dissection. In: Scarci M, Solli P, Sihoe AD, editors. Minimally invasive thoracic surgery: principles and practice of thoracoscopic technique. London: JP Medical; 2017. p. 37–40.

8 Prevention and Management of Complications During Video-Assisted Thoracic Surgery Lung Resection and Lymph Node Dissection

Yong Soo Choi

Abstract

Intraoperative events can occur during video-assisted thoracoscopic surgery (VATS) lobectomy due to unfavorable surgical anatomy, such as dense adhesions or calcifications around the pulmonary arteries. Troubleshooting intraoperative complications is essential for performing safe and successful VATS pulmonary resection and lymph node dissection. If continuous bleeding occurs or VATS does not proceed despite all measures, conversion to open thoracotomy should not be delayed.

Keywords

Video-assisted thoracoscopic surgery
Intraoperative events · Complication

8.1 Introduction

Video-assisted thoracoscopic surgery (VATS) pulmonary resection and lymph node dissection is a widely accepted technique for early-stage non-small cell lung cancer [1, 2]. A learning curve is required to perform VATS lobectomy for lung cancer. VATS lobectomy is known to be associated with a significantly higher rate of intraoperative complications than open thoracotomy lobectomy [3]. Intraoperative events can occur during VATS lobectomy when performed by either an experienced surgeon or a novice surgeon due to unfavorable surgical anatomy, such as dense adhesions or calcifications around the pulmonary arteries. Troubleshooting intraoperative complications is essential for performing safe and successful VATS pulmonary resection and lymph node dissection. This article reviews the causes, related factors, and troubleshooting and prevention strategies for intraoperative events during VATS.

8.2 Bleeding

Significant unexpected bleeding mainly occurs due to injuries of the pulmonary arteries, pulmonary veins, and bronchial arteries. Inappropriate and unclear exposure and careless dissection, ligation, or division of vessel structures were found to be the most common causes of vascular injuries [4]. Stapler or device malfunction leading to bleeding is relatively rare, and most cases are likely related to the surgeon's error [5].

The most common bleeding sites during VATS are the pulmonary arteries. It is recognized that patients receiving neoadjuvant chemotherapy and/or radiation therapy and those with larger tumors are at greater risk for an arterial injury [6, 7]. The presence of calcified lymph nodes

Y. S. Choi (✉)
Department of Thoracic and Cardiovascular Surgery, Samsung Medical Center, Sungkyunkwan University School of Medicine, Seoul, Republic of Korea
e-mail: ysooyah.choi@samsung.com

K. Kim et al. (eds.), *Techniques in Minimally Invasive Thoracic Surgery*,
https://doi.org/10.1007/978-981-19-2472-9_8

between the pulmonary artery and bronchus causes bleeding issues, especially in older patients with previous inflammatory disease. Pulmonary vein injuries are much less common than pulmonary artery injuries. Careless dissection of the inferior pulmonary ligament can cause injuries to the inferior pulmonary vein. Bleeding from the bronchial arteries is common during VATS, but can be easily controlled by compression, electrocautery, ultrasonic energy devices, or hemoclips. However, postoperative bleeding from the bronchial arteries, especially along the bronchial stump or subcarinal area, requires reoperation for bleeding control.

Appropriate exposure and detection of anatomical structures with attention to careful and meticulous vascular dissection, ligation, and division are the most critical elements for avoiding serious injuries [8]. Inadequate exposure of the hilar structures is rather common when vision is provided from the lower port below the sixth intercostal space. Three-dimensional VATS provides better visualization than two-dimensional VATS [9, 10], enabling more comfortable identification and dissection of vascular structures.

A basic safety strategy is to keep a sponge or a clamp on the back table as preparation for sudden unexpected bleeding during any minimally invasive surgery. The instant goal is the immediate control of hemorrhage and restoring the view of the operative field. Direct compression using a sponge stick or the surrounding lung is an effective way to stop or decrease bleeding from injured vessels. However, in cases of massive bleeding, it may not be easy to identify the bleeding focus. After sufficient compression for at least a few minutes, while maintaining a stable blood pressure and heart rate, the decision should be made regarding how to control bleeding and continue with the next step of the procedure. Conversion to open thoracotomy should also be considered if the vital signs are unstable due to continuous bleeding. Compression itself, electrocautery, hemostatic clips, and other hemostatic agents may also be used. A wet fibrin sealant patch is placed over the bleeding focus and compressed gently for at least a few minutes. This maneuver is usually enough to stop bleeding. If bleeding continues, vascular clamping of the proximal portion of the bleeding focus with an endoscopic vascular clamp is the next step, but it is difficult for novice surgeons to control the bleeding with a vascular clamp. After successfully clamping the proximal part of the injured vessel, primary repair with a suture could be done. Increasing the number of VATS ports may be helpful to obtain better exposure of the injured vessels and control the bleeding.

A novel method for managing vascular injuries, called the suction–compression angiorrhaphy technique, involves first controlling bleeding by side-compression of the injured site with endoscopic suction. Then, angiorrhaphy is performed with a running suture, with the specific procedure depending on the size and location of the injuries; options include direct suturing upon suction compression, suturing after substituting suction compression with clamping of the injured site, or suturing after attaining proximal cross-clamping of the main pulmonary artery [11].

If bleeding continues despite all measures, conversion to open thoracotomy should not be delayed. Compression with a sponge stick over the bleeding focus should be maintained via the lower port when making the thoracotomy extension.

8.3 Bronchus Injury, Fused Interlobar Fissure, and Air Leak

Bronchial injuries occurred in 6 (0.94%) of 633 patients who underwent VATS anatomic lung resection, requiring 3 unplanned pneumonectomies and 1 unplanned bilobectomy, and causing 1 tracheoesophageal fistula and 1 membranous airway injury to the bronchus intermedius [3]. Direct injury to the bronchus by electrocautery or an ultrasonic device is clearly identified during the air leak test after the completion of lung resection, but it is not possible to check intraoperatively for a delayed bronchial injury caused by a thermal mechanism. A minimal injury to the membranous portion of the bronchus or an inadequately stapled stump of the bronchus can become aggravated to form a bronchopleural fistula in patients with diabetes mellitus or chronic steroid usage. Reinforcement of the bronchial stump with pericardium or a fibrin sealant patch over the bronchial stump and neighboring bronchus could decrease the risk of bronchial fistula after the operation.

When lobectomy is performed in a patient with a fused interlobar fissure, there is a higher risk of air leakage [12]. There is no consensus regarding the choice between a fissure-last technique [13] and a fissure-first technique [14] during VATS lobectomy. Careful identification of the pulmonary vein pathway is required in cases of right upper lobectomy. Some portions of the middle lobe and lower lobe drained into the superior pulmonary vein via the upper pulmonary vein, so careless transection of those tributaries may result in congestion of the middle lobe and lower lobe after right upper lobectomy. Therefore, a fissure-first technique is recommended in right upper lobectomy. A totally fused, thick interlobar fissure is a reason for conversion to open thoracotomy.

Prolonged air leak is a major reason for long hospital stays and remains a common complication after VATS lobectomy. Several risk factors for prolonged air leak have been identified, including old age, a body mass index under 24.0 kg/m^2, the surgeon's experience, the surgical site (upper lobectomy and bilobectomy), decreased pulmonary function, fused fissure, and pleural adhesions [15, 16]. Meticulous care should be taken during the division of a fused fissure and pleural adhesiolysis in patients with these factors.

8.4 Miscellaneous Tips to Manage and Prevent Intraoperative Events

1. Postoperative delayed gastric emptying could be minimized by taking care not to damage the vagus nerve, especially when dissecting the subcarinal nodes and aortopulmonary nodes. Meticulous care should be taken when performing lobectomy and node dissection in patients who have previously undergone contralateral lobectomy and node dissection.
2. Avoid damaging the recurrent laryngeal nerve when dissecting the right upper paratracheal nodes and left lower paratracheal nodes and aortopulmonary nodes.
3. Injuries of the diaphragm or esophagus are indolent and subclinical during the operation or the immediate postoperative days.
4. The anvil tip of endoscopic staplers is slightly traumatic, so care should be taken when manipulating staplers.
5. Conversion to open thoracotomy should not be considered a source of shame to the surgeon. Even experts need to convert to thoracotomy when facing a difficult situation during VATS lobectomy. Please do not forget that VATS is not a goal of surgery itself, but instead one of multiple approach techniques.Conflict of InterestNo potential conflict of interest relevant to this article was reported.

References

1. Ettinger DS, Akerley W, Borghaei H, et al. Non-small cell lung cancer, version 2.2013. J Natl Compr Canc Netw. 2013;11:645–53.
2. Gopaldas RR, Bakaeen FG, Dao TK, Walsh GL, Swisher SG, Chu D. Video-assisted thoracoscopic versus open thoracotomy lobectomy in a cohort of 13,619 patients. Ann Thorac Surg. 2010;89:1563–70.
3. Flores RM, Ihekweazu U, Dycoco J, et al. Video-assisted thoracoscopic surgery (VATS) lobectomy: catastrophic intraoperative complications. J Thorac Cardiovasc Surg. 2011;142:1412–7.
4. Louie BE. Catastrophes and complicated intraoperative events during robotic lung resection. J Visc Surg. 2017;3:52.
5. Brown SL, Woo EK. Surgical stapler-associated fatalities and adverse events reported to the Food and Drug Administration. J Am Coll Surg. 2004;199:374–81.
6. Decaluwe H, Petersen RH, Hansen H, et al. Major intraoperative complications during video-assisted thoracoscopic anatomical lung resections: an intention-to-treat analysis. Eur J Cardiothorac Surg. 2015;48:588–99.
7. Augustin F, Maier HT, Weissenbacher A, et al. Causes, predictors and consequences of conversion from VATS to open lung lobectomy. Surg Endosc. 2016;30:2415–21.

8. Safdie FM, Sanchez MV, Sarkaria IS. Prevention and management of intraoperative crisis in VATS and open chest surgery: how to avoid emergency conversion. J Visc Surg. 2017;3:87.
9. Dong S, Yang XN, Zhong WZ, et al. Comparison of three-dimensional and two-dimensional visualization in video-assisted thoracoscopic lobectomy. Thorac Cancer. 2016;7:530–4.
10. Kim TH, Hong TH, Choi YS. Comparison of surgical outcomes between 3D and 2D VATS lobectomy for clinical stage I lung cancer. Precis Future Med. 2020;4:69–74.
11. Mei J, Pu Q, Liao H, Ma L, Zhu Y, Liu L. A novel method for troubleshooting vascular injury during anatomic thoracoscopic pulmonary resection without conversion to thoracotomy. Surg Endosc. 2013;27:530–7.
12. Igai H, Kamiyoshihara M, Yoshikawa R, et al. The efficacy of thoracoscopic fissureless lobectomy in patients with dense fissures. J Thorac Dis. 2016;8:3691–6.
13. Balsara KR, Balderson SS, D'Amico TA. Surgical techniques to avoid parenchymal injury during lung resection (fissureless lobectomy). Thorac Surg Clin. 2010;20:365–9.
14. Decaluwe H, Sokolow Y, Deryck F, et al. Thoracoscopic tunnel technique for anatomical lung resections: a 'fissure first, hilum last' approach with staplers in the fissureless patient. Interact Cardiovasc Thorac Surg. 2015;21:2–7.
15. Rivera C, Bernard A, Falcoz PE, et al. Characterization and prediction of prolonged air leak after pulmonary resection: a nationwide study setting up the index of prolonged air leak. Ann Thorac Surg. 2011;92:1062–8.
16. Zhao K, Mei J, Xia C, et al. Prolonged air leak after video-assisted thoracic surgery lung cancer resection: risk factors and its effect on postoperative clinical recovery. J Thorac Dis. 2017;9:1219–25.

Robot-Assisted Thoracic Surgery in Non-Small Cell Lung Cancer

9

Jun Hee Lee, Kook Nam Han, and Hyun Koo Kim

Abstract

Lobectomy is the standard treatment for early non-small cell lung cancer. Various surgical techniques for lobectomy have been developed, and minimally invasive thoracic surgery, such as video-assisted thoracic surgery or robot-assisted thoracic surgery, has been considered as an alternative to conventional open thoracotomy. Recently, Robotic lobectomy is becoming increasingly popular since the first case series was published in 2002. Several studies have reported that robotic lobectomy has comparable oncologic and perioperative outcomes to those of video-assisted thoracic surgery lobectomy and open lobectomy. However, robotic lobectomy remains a challenge for surgeons because of the steep learning curve, reduced tactile sensation, difficulty in port placement, and challenges in cooperation between the surgeon and assistant. Many studies have reported on robotic lobectomy, but few have presented surgical techniques for robotic lobectomy. In this article, the surgical techniques and optimal performance of robotic lobectomy are described in detail for all five types of lobectomy for surgeons beginning with robotic lobectomy.

J. H. Lee · K. N. Han
Department of Thoracic and Cardiovascular Surgery, Korea University Guro Hospital, Korea University College of Medicine, Seoul, Republic of Korea

H. K. Kim (✉)
Thoracic and Cardiovascular Surgery, Korea University Guro Hospital, Seoul, Republic of Korea
e-mail: kimhyunkoo@korea.ac.kr

Keywords

Robot-assisted thoracic surgery · Robotic lobectomy · Lobectomy · Lung neoplasms

9.1 Introduction

Lobectomy, which involves the anatomical resection of an entire lobe of the lung, is the standard treatment for early non-small cell lung cancer (NSCLC). Traditionally, it was performed via an open thoracotomy approach, which is associated with severe postoperative pain and a large wound. Minimally invasive thoracic surgery lobectomy, including video-assisted thoracic surgery (VATS) and robotic lobectomy, has been considered an appropriate approach and is associated with low perioperative morbidity, less pain, shorter hospitalization, and equivalent oncologic outcomes compared with open thoracotomy [1–5].

Since the first report of VATS lobectomy in the early 1990s [6], it has become a popular surgical approach [7–9]. However, several disadvantages of VATS lobectomy, such as the lack of flexibility, difficulty of hand–eye coordination, and limitations of two-dimensional imaging, led to the development of robotic lobectomy as a

K. Kim et al. (eds.), *Techniques in Minimally Invasive Thoracic Surgery*,
https://doi.org/10.1007/978-981-19-2472-9_9

novel technique [10]. Robotic lobectomy, which is performed with a robotic surgical system, offers improved three-dimensional imaging, hand–eye coordination, freedom of movement, and tremor filtration, allowing safe surgical procedures [11, 12].

Since the first case series on robotic lobectomy, reported in 2002 [13], it has gradually developed with technological innovations of robotic systems. The introduction of a robotic stapler (EndoWrist Stapler; Intuitive Surgical Inc., Sunnyvale, CA, USA) in the da Vinci Xi has made it possible for total robotic lobectomy to be directly controlled by surgeons, and may reduce the operative time [12, 14, 15].

Several studies have reported the advantages of robotic lobectomy, which is associated with a significant reduction in the length of hospitalization, chest tube drainage duration, postoperative complications, and mortality when compared with the open thoracotomy approach [2, 16–19]. Two studies using propensity score matching for the outcomes of open, VATS, and robotic lobectomy demonstrated no significant differences in morbidity and oncologic outcomes [20, 21].

In recent years, robotic lobectomy has been indicated for more challenging cases owing to its superior maneuverability. Qiu et al. [22] reported a successful case of robotic double-sleeve lobectomy and demonstrated its ability to be used for bronchoplasty and angioplasty. Wilson et al. [23] reported the prevalence of nodal upstaging during robotic lobectomy in early NSCLC; therefore, robotic mediastinal lymph node dissection (MLND) may be useful in patients with locally advanced N2 NSCLC due to improved dexterity and visualization.

However, robotic lobectomy remains a challenge because of its steep learning curve, reduced tactile sensation, difficulty in port placement, and challenges in cooperation between the surgeon and assistant. Robotic lobectomy techniques have many variations in terms of the number of incisions, number of robotic arms used, use of a utility incision, site location for port placement, and use of CO_2 insufflation. These variations add to the difficulty of the procedure.

In this article, the surgical techniques and optimal performance of robot lobectomy are described in detail for all five types of lobectomy for surgeons beginning to perform robotic lobectomy, along with useful tips on how to overcome procedure-related problems.

9.2 Indications and Contraindications of Robotic Surgery

The indications for robotic lobectomy are similar to those for conventional lobectomy, although they may be more extensive than those of VATS and open lobectomy. Robotic lobectomy may be indicated in patients with marginal pulmonary function and locally advanced cancer [24, 25]. Generally, some conditions such as dense adhesions, bronchial invasion, chest wall invasion, hilar nodal invasion, preoperative radiotherapy, prior thoracic surgery, and hilar nodal invasion are no longer regarded as absolute contraindications; instead, they are considered relative contraindication [4, 26]. In our opinion, robotic lobectomy by an experienced surgeon is feasible in these patients.

9.3 Learning Curve of Robotic Surgery

Although defining the learning curve is difficult, several studies have estimated the learning curve for a robotic lobectomy to be 18–32 cases (Table 9.1). According to some studies, at least 20 cases are required for surgical competence [18, 27, 28]. Arnold et al. [29] reported a learning curve of 22 cases, while Song et al. [30] reported it as 32 cases for the surgeon and 20 cases for the bedside assistant.

Few studies have compared the learning curves of robotic lobectomy and VATS lobectomy. Jang et al. [31] reported the outcomes of their experiences of performing robotic lobectomy with VATS lobectomy. They compared the outcomes of their early experience of robotic

Table 9.1 The learning curve in robotic lobectomy

Study	Year	Surgical technique	Total no. of patients who underwent robotic lobectomy	No. of operations required to achieve surgical competence
Melfi and Mussi [27]	2008	4 ports, 4 arms	107	20
Gharagozloo et al. [28]	2009	3 ports, 3 arms	100	20
Veronesi et al. [18]	2010	4 ports, 4 arms	54	20
Arnold et al. [29]	2019	5 ports, 4 arms	101	22
Song et al. [30]	2019	4 ports, 3 arms	208	32 (for surgeon) 20 (for assistant)

lobectomy ($n = 40$) with the outcomes of initial ($n = 40$) and recent VATS lobectomy ($n = 40$). The complication rates (10% versus 32.5%, $p = 0.027$), intraoperative bleeding (219 mL versus 374 mL, $p = 0.017$), and the median length of postoperative stay (6 days versus 9 days, $p < 0.001$) was significantly lower in the robotic lobectomy group than in the initial VATS group.

In the future, robotic surgery training programs consisting of simulated skills training, dry lab-based learning, and video articles can help shorten this learning curve.

9.4 Operative Technique

General Considerations

A double-lumen tube is placed for 1-lung ventilation, and the patient is positioned in the lateral decubitus position. The operating table is flexed to widen the intercostal space (ICS) and to move the hip down. If possible, the patients are placed in the reverse Trendelenburg position. Port mapping is performed according to the use of the utility incision, the location of the lobe to be resected, and the number of ports required. After an appropriate incision, the robotic trocar and working port are placed. In patients with a narrow thoracic cavity or short stature, a single port with multi-instrument access (Lapsingle; Sejong Medical, Paju, Korea) is used at our center with CO_2 insufflation (maximum 6–10 mmHg), which facilitates lung collapse and caudal shift of the diaphragm.

Before robot docking, a careful thoracoscopic examination is required to identify the pleural adhesion, pleural effusions, and other metastases. We routinely place the vessel loop and rolled-up gauze in the fissure before the introduction of instrument arms to save time (Fig. 9.1a). The use of a vessel loop for retraction of the vessel branches and bronchus facilitates stapling and prevents vascular injury (Fig. 9.1b). The placement of rolled-up gauze between the robot wrist and the structure that needs to be retracted facilitates dissection without the fourth robotic arm or the assistant at the bedside, especially for the hilar and nodal tissues (Fig. 9.1c).

The robotic endoscope is always installed centrally, and other devices are installed depending on the surgeon's preference. A Cadiere grasper is installed on the left, and a Maryland bipolar forceps is installed on the right. Most vessels, as well as the bronchi, are divided with the robotic stapler (EndoWrist Stapler; Intuitive Surgical Inc., Sunnyvale, CA, USA) in the da Vinci Xi surgical system, and small vessel branches can be ligated with robotic Hem-o-Lok clips.

Robotic MLND is routinely performed in all patients. Complete dissection of the hilar lymph nodes is a key point in robotic lobectomy. It is always optimal to remove all nodal tissues around and among hilar structures, because doing so helps to identify the anatomy and removing these nodal tissues makes it easy to pass through the stapler. The cut end of the surgical glove is used as a retrieval bag, and the resected lymph nodes are retrieved at the cut end of the surgical glove to

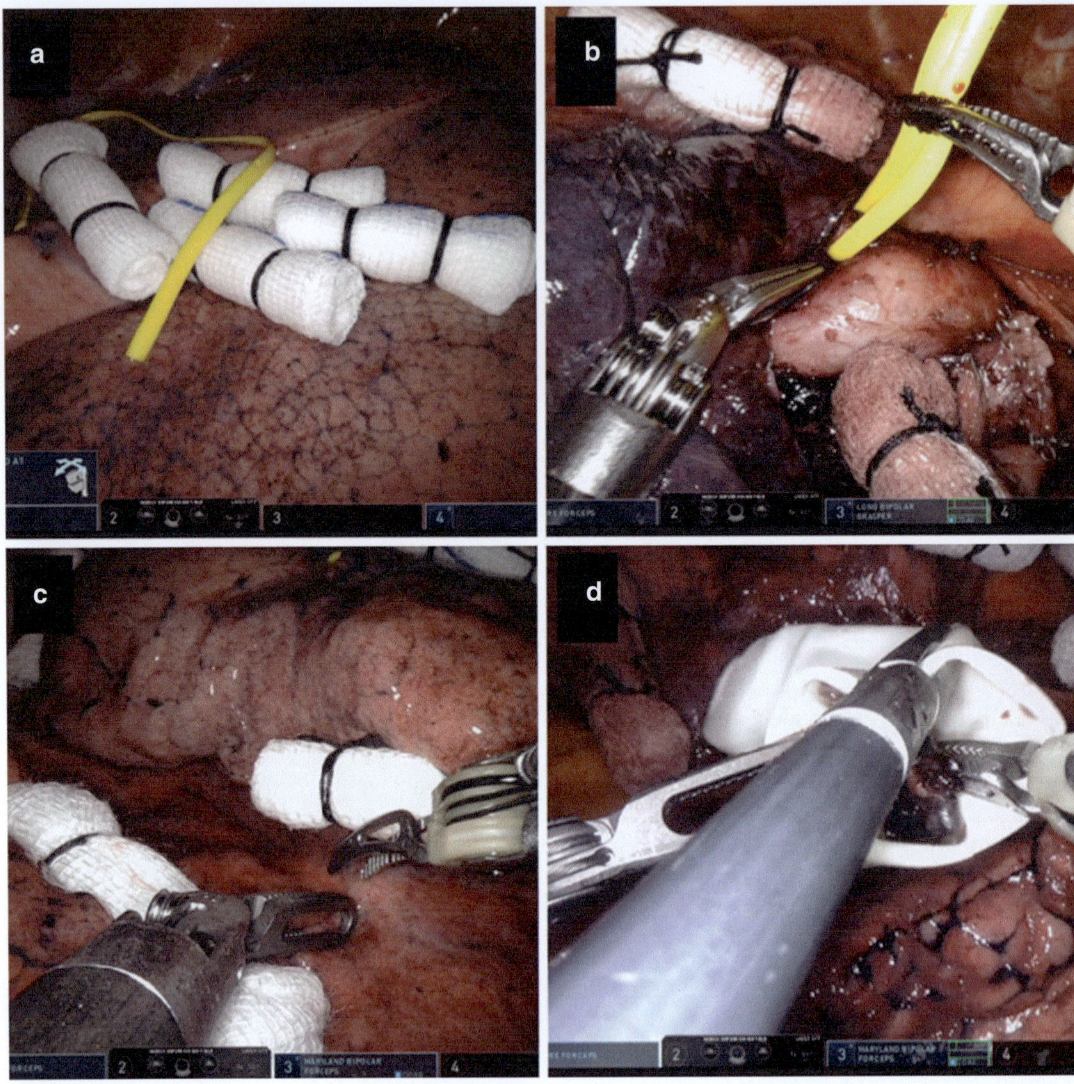

Fig. 9.1 Tips for robotic lobectomy. (**a**) Placement of rolled-up gauze and a vessel loop on the fissure. (**b**) Pulmonary artery isolated with a vessel loop. (**c**) Surgical field with traction using rolled gauze. (**d**) The cut end of the surgical glove as a retrieval bag for the resected lymph nodes

avoid contamination of the wound and thoracic cavity with cancer cells (Fig. 9.1d).

At the end of the procedure, the lung specimens are removed using a specimen bag through the utility incision. We routinely perform a paravertebral intercostal nerve block, which is an intrapleural administration of bupivacaine via the intrathoracic approach under endoscopic visualization. Before closing the wound incision, a 24 F or 20 F chest tube is inserted into the incision.

Port Mapping

Optimal port placement is a vitally important component of the success of robotic lobectomy, as it avoids compression injuries, allows free mobility of the robotic instruments, and facilitates safe surgery. Currently, robotic lobectomy is performed using 3–4 arms with 2–4 ports, with the exception that a few surgeons use the 5-port approach. When using a robotic stapler, creating a 12-mm port for the stapler as low as possible can facilitate robotic arm maneuverability, because the end effector of the robotic stapler is longer than the other robotic instruments [32].

The 4-Port Approach

Veronesi et al. [18] and Pardolesi et al. [33] introduced 4-port robotic lobectomy, consisting of 3 trocar ports and 1 utility port. A 3- to 4-cm utility incision is made at the fifth ICS anterior to the latissimus dorsi. A 12-mm port incision (camera port) is made in the seventh ICS at the midaxillary line for right-side lobectomy, while the incision site is 2 cm posterior for left-side lobectomy. An 8-mm port incision is made at the eighth ICS 8 cm posteriorly from the camera port, and the other 8-mm port incision is made in the auscultatory triangle [18, 33].

Cerfolio et al. [34] introduced 4-port robotic lobectomy consisting of 3 ports and 1 assistant port. One 5-mm port incision (videoscope) is made at the sixth or seventh ICS along the midaxillary line, and another 5-mm port incision (robotic arm 3) is made at the seventh to eighth ICS, just anterior to the spinous process of the vertebral body. An 8-mm port (robotic arm 2) is made at the seventh to eighth ICS, 10 cm anterior to robotic arm 3. The camera port is made at the seventh to eighth ICS, 9 cm anterior to robotic arm 2. A 15-mm assistant port is made at the 2 or 3 lower ribs [34].

The 3-Port Approach

A 3- to 4-cm utility incision is made at the seventh or eighth ICS along the midaxillary line, a 12-mm port incision is made at the sixth or seventh ICS along the anterior axillary line, and the other 12-mm port incision is made at the eighth or ninth ICS along the scapular line, 8 cm apart from each other. A single port with multi-instrument access (Lapsingle; Sejong Medical) is installed through the utility incision. An 8-mm trocar for the robotic camera is inserted through the working port, and the assistant inserts his or her instruments through the other side of the working port (Fig. 9.2).

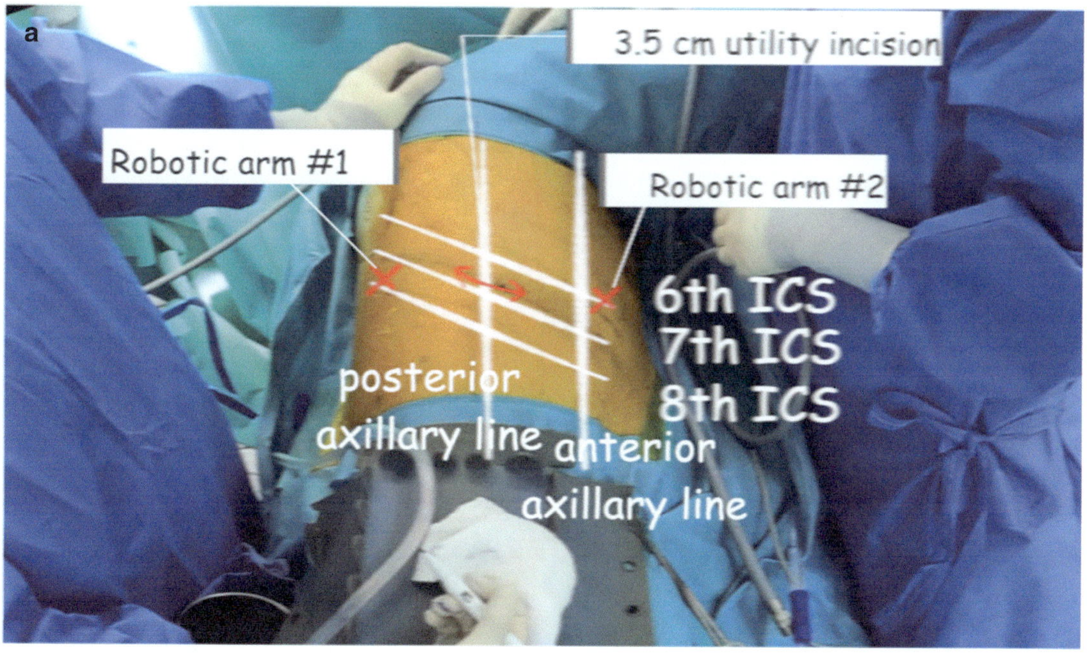

Fig. 9.2 (**a–c**) Photographs of port placement in the 3-port approach for robotic lobectomy. *ICS* intercostal space

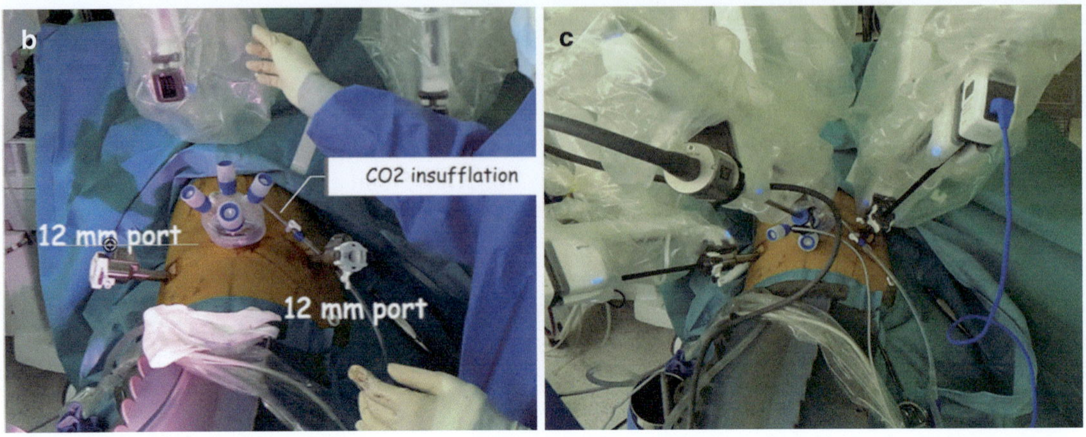

Fig. 9.2 (continued)

The 2-Port Approach

A 3- to 4-cm utility incision (camera and arm port 2) is made at the seventh or eighth ICS, along the posterior axillary line, and a 12-mm port incision (arm port 1) is made at the sixth or seventh ICS along the anterior axillary line without an assistant port. A single port with multi-instrument access (Lapsingle; Sejong Medical) is installed through the utility incision. Two 8-mm trocars for the robotic camera and robotic arm 1 (for a Cadiere grasper or Maryland bipolar forceps) are inserted through the working port. The 12-mm trocars are inserted through another 12-mm port for robotic arm 2 (Cadiere grasper, Maryland bipolar forceps, or robotic EndoWrist staplers). The assistant inserts his or her instruments through the space between two trocars in the working port (Fig. 9.3).

The Five Types of Lobectomy

Below are descriptions of how to perform each type of lobectomy.

Right Upper Lobectomy

The dissection of the hilar structures should be performed individually, and lymphadenectomy should also be performed. The anatomical structures are carefully identified (especially in the posterior ascending artery). The surgical approach differs depending on the completeness of the pulmonary fissure.

When the fissure is fused and not well developed, the hilar approach is preferred to dissect the mediastinal pleura over the anterior hilum. The sequence of dissection is anterior to posterior in a single direction, as shown in Fig. 9.4: (1) isolation and division of the right upper lobe (RUL) vein, (2) isolation and division of the anterior trunk of the pulmonary artery, (3) isolation and division of posterior ascending artery, (4) isolation and division of the RUL bronchus, and (5) completion of the fissure. The sequence of steps 1 and 2 can be changed.

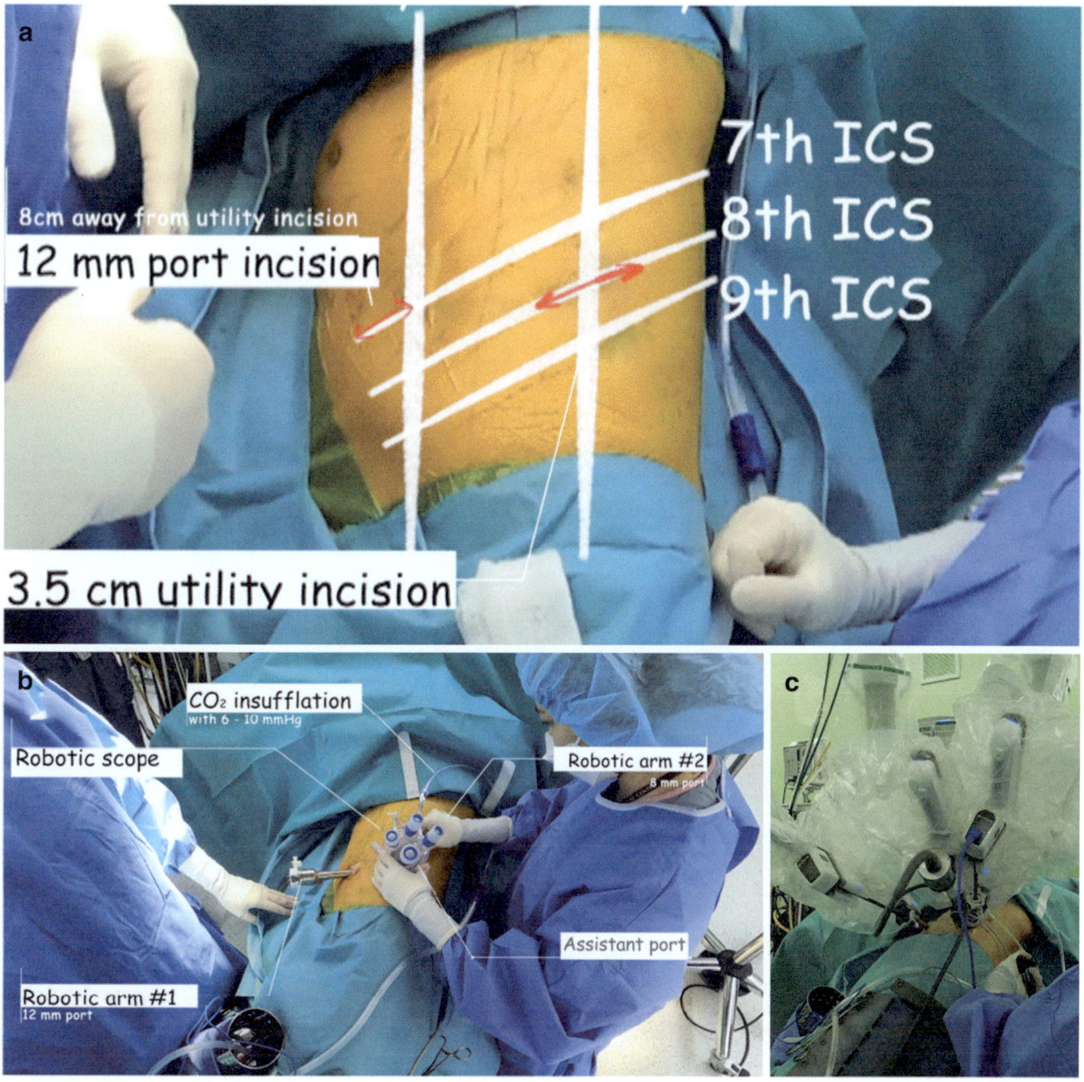

Fig. 9.3 (**a–c**) Photographs of port placement in the 2-port approach for robotic lobectomy. *ICS* intercostal space

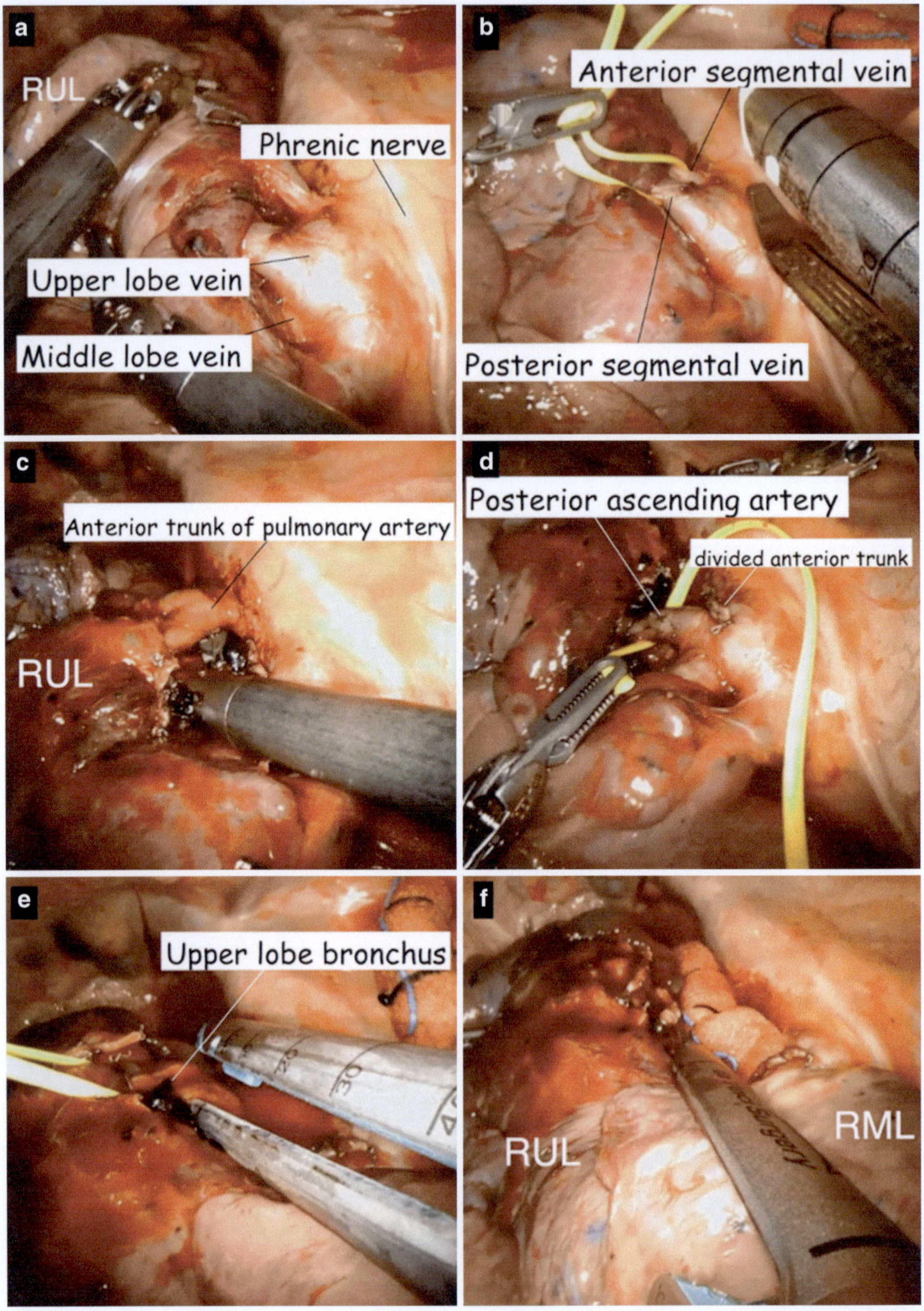

Fig. 9.4 Robotic right upper lobectomy for patients with a fused fissure. (**a**) Identification of the bifurcation between the middle lobe vein and upper lobe vein. (**b**) Division of the upper lobe vein. (**c**) Isolation of the anterior trunk of the pulmonary artery. (**d**) Isolation of the posterior ascending artery. (**e**) Division of the upper lobe bronchus. (**f**) Completion of the fissure. *RUL* right upper lobe, *RML* right middle lobe

Step 1: Isolation and Division of the RUL Vein

The RUL is retracted posteriorly to expose the upper hilar region and the anterior mediastinum, and the anterior mediastinum and anterior mediastinal pleura are opened to expose the upper lobe vein. Once the upper lobe vein is identified, dissection is continued until the bifurcation between the middle lobe vein and upper lobe vein is identified. The anterior segmental vein and posterior segmental vein are encircled with a vessel loop and divided with a robotic stapler.

Step 2: Isolation and Division of the Anterior Trunk of the Pulmonary Artery

After division of the upper lobe vein, the hilum is carefully dissected to expose the pulmonary artery. The connective tissue and nodal tissue around the pulmonary artery are removed to expose the anterior trunk of the pulmonary artery. The anterior trunk is isolated from the main pulmonary artery, and the grasper is passed behind the anterior trunk to ensure sufficient space for the stapler's passage. The anterior trunk of the pulmonary artery is encircled with a vessel loop and divided using a robotic stapler.

Step 3: Isolation and Division of the Posterior Ascending Artery

Division of the posterior ascending artery can be performed before or after division of the RUL bronchus. The posterior ascending artery is encircled with a vessel loop and divided with robotic stapler. When the posterior ascending artery is too small, robotic Hem-o-Lok clips can be used to ligate it.

Step 4: Isolation and Division of the RUL Bronchus

Complete dissection of the lymph nodes should be performed, which facilitates the passage of the stapler. The upper lobe is retracted anteriorly, and the posterior aspect of the hilum is dissected. The dissection is continued to expose the RUL bronchus and bronchus intermedius. The upper lobe bronchus is encircled with a vessel loop and divided with a robotic stapler.

Step 5: Completion of the Fissure

To complete the fissure, it is usually divided with a robotic stapler. Care is taken to identify the main pulmonary artery and right middle lobe (RML) artery. Next, the specimen is removed using a specimen bag through the utility incision.

However, when the fissure is complete and well developed, we prefer to perform the steps in the following order (Fig. 9.5): (1) isolation and division of the posterior ascending artery, (2) dissection of the pleura at the RUL bronchus and bronchus intermedius bifurcation, (3) isolation and division of the anterior trunk of the pulmo-

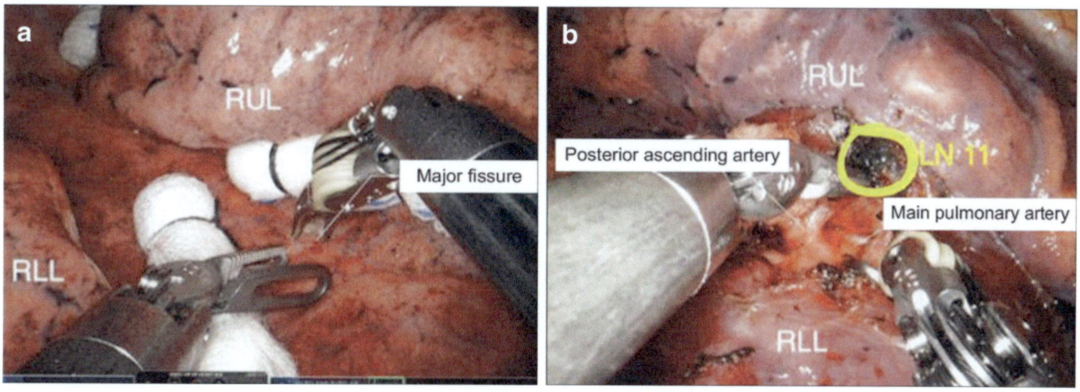

Fig. 9.5 Robotic right upper lobectomy for patients with a complete fissure. (**a**) Dissection of the major fissure. (**b**) Identification of the posterior ascending artery. (**c**) Dissection of the pleura at the right upper lobe (RUL) bronchus and bronchus intermedius bifurcation. (**d**) Division of the posterior ascending artery. (**e**) Identification of the anterior trunk of pulmonary artery and superior pulmonary vein. (**f**) Division of the anterior trunk of pulmonary artery. (**g**) Division of the upper lobe bronchus. (**h**) Division of the upper lobe vein. *LN* lymph node

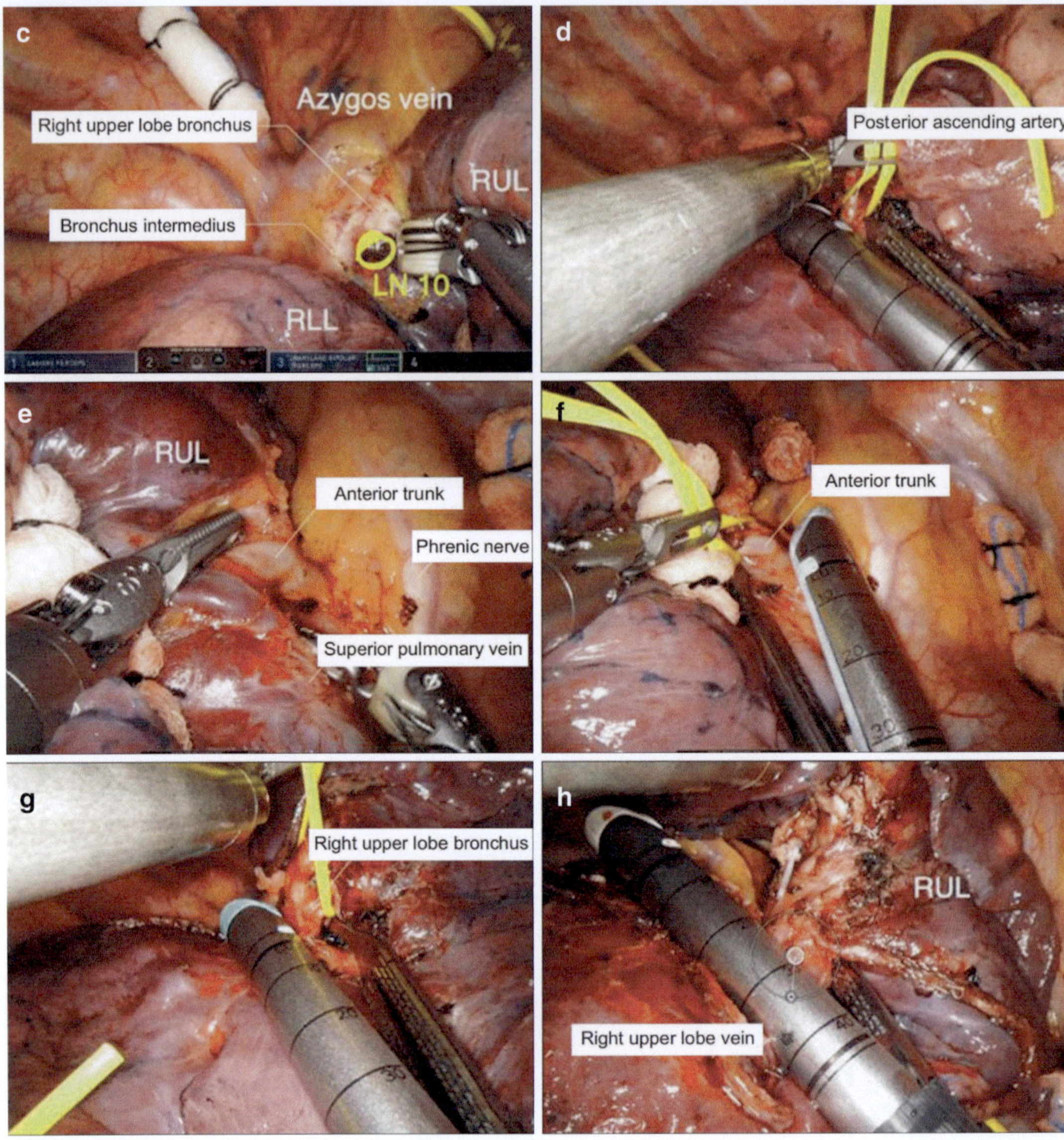

Fig. 9.5 (continued)

nary artery, (4) isolation and division of the RUL bronchus, and (5) isolation and division of the RUL vein.

Step 1: Isolation and Division of the Posterior Ascending Artery

The RUL is retracted superiorly, and the right lower lobe (RLL) is retracted inferiorly to expose the pulmonary artery. The major fissure between the RUL and RLL is dissected using long bipolar forceps, and the nodal tissues are removed to identify the anatomy of the pulmonary artery. Once the posterior ascending artery is exposed, the dissection continues until the main pulmonary artery is identified. The incomplete major fissure between the RUL and RLL can be divided with a robotic stapler to expose the pulmonary artery. Sometimes it is better to divide the major fissure last to reduce air leakage. The posterior ascending artery is encircled with a vessel loop and divided using a robotic stapler. If the posterior ascending artery is too small, robotic Hem-o-Lok clips can be used to ligate it.

Step 2: Dissection of the Pleura at the RUL Bronchus and Bronchus Intermedius Bifurcation

The lung is retracted inferiorly to expose the superior surface of the hilum, and the upper hilar region is dissected. This prepares the field for the isolation of the RUL bronchus. Once the connective and nodal tissues are removed, the right main bronchus and the bronchus intermedius are clearly exposed.

Step 3: Isolation and Division of the Anterior Trunk of the Pulmonary Artery

The lung is retracted posteriorly, and the upper hilar region is dissected anteriorly to posteriorly. Once the anterior trunk is exposed, it should be separated from the superior pulmonary vein. The anterior trunk is encircled with a vessel loop and divided using a robotic stapler.

Step 4: Isolation and Division of the RUL Bronchus

After division of the anterior trunk, the RUL bronchus is exposed, and nodal tissues around the bronchus should be removed. The RUL bronchus is encircled with a vessel loop and divided using a robotic stapler.

Step 5: Isolation and Division of the RUL Vein

The bifurcation between the RML vein and upper lobe vein should be dissected to identify anomalies of the venous anatomy. Before division of the RUL vein, the incomplete minor fissure between the RUL and RML is usually divided using a robotic stapler. The RUL is retracted superiorly, and the RUL vein is divided using a robotic stapler. Next, the specimen is removed using a specimen bag via the utility incision.

Right Middle Lobectomy

Although there are many variations in the techniques of right middle robotic lobectomy, we prefer to perform the procedure in the following order (Fig. 9.6): (1) division of the major fissure, (2) division of the middle lobe vein, (3) division of the middle lobe bronchus, (4) division of the middle lobe artery, and (5) division of the minor fissure.

Complete dissection of the hilar lymph nodes is the key element of robotic right middle lobectomy because of the narrow space between structures, and it facilitates the identification of the

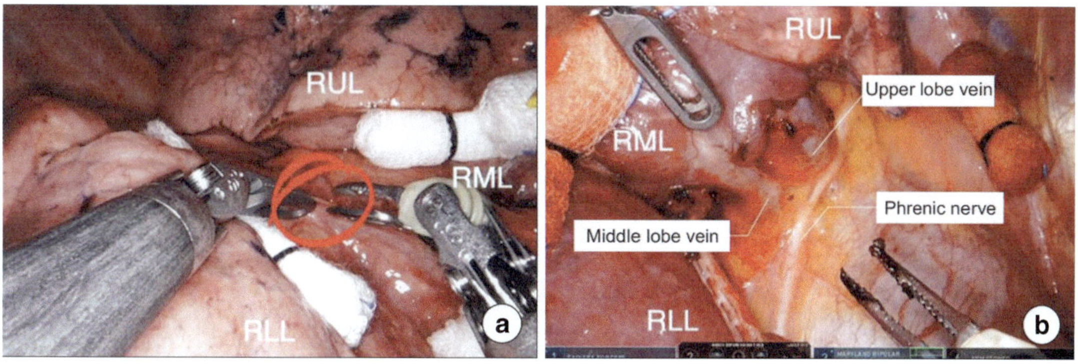

Fig. 9.6 Robotic right middle lobectomy. (**a**) Dissection of the major fissure. (**b**) Identification of the bifurcation between the middle lobe vein and upper lobe vein. (**c**) Division of the middle lobe vein. (**d**) Division of the middle lobe bronchus. (**e**) Division of the middle lobe artery. (**f**) Completion of the minor fissure. *RUL* right upper lobe, *RML* right middle lobe, *RLL* right lower lobe, *PA* pulmonary artery

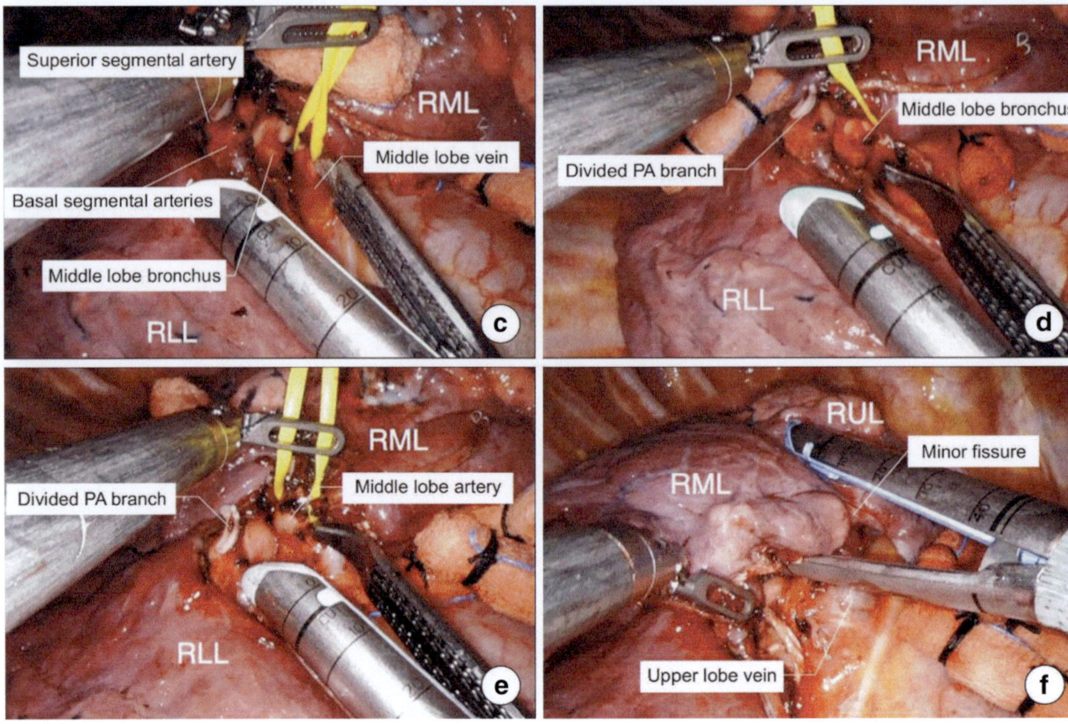

Fig. 9.6 (continued)

middle lobe bronchus and middle lobe artery. The phrenic nerve is carefully identified.

Step 1: Dissection and Division of the Major Fissure

We usually prefer to dissect the anterior portion of the major fissure first with long bipolar forceps. The interlobar lymph nodes are carefully removed to facilitate the identification of the pulmonary artery, bronchus, and vein. Once the artery to the RLL is identified, a tunnel for the division of the major fissure can be created. Part of the incomplete major fissure can be divided using a robotic stapler.

Step 2: Isolation and Division of the RML Vein

Once the major fissure is divided, the pulmonary vein is well exposed. After retraction of the lung posteriorly, the anterior aspect of the hilum is dissected. Although the middle lobe vein most often joins the superior pulmonary vein, it may join the right inferior pulmonary vein and directly drain into the atrium. After identification of the RUL vein and RML vein, the RML vein is encircled with a vessel loop and divided with a robotic stapler.

Step 3: Isolation and Division of the Middle Lobar Bronchus

The middle lobe bronchus is always located below the middle lobe artery. The middle lobe bronchus is dissected and complete dissection of the lymph node should be performed before closing and dividing by the stapler. The middle lobar bronchus is encircled with a vessel loop and divided using a robotic stapler. After clamping the bronchus and before firing the stapler, ventilation of the right lung can confirm the exact position of the stapler. The minor fissure can be divided using a robotic stapler before or after division of the middle lobe artery.

Step 4: Isolation and Division of the Middle Lobe Artery

The nodal tissues should be dissected completely to identify the anatomy of the pulmonary artery. A4 and A5 can arise as separate branches (in 50% of cases) or a common trunk (in the other 50% of cases) from the interlobar artery. The middle lobe artery is encircled with a vessel loop and divided using a robotic stapler. Once all the hilar structures are divided, the minor fissure between the RUL and RML is usually divided using a robotic stapler. Next, the specimen is removed using a specimen bag via the utility incision.

Right Lower Lobectomy

The inferior pulmonary ligament is usually dissected first to approach the inferior pulmonary vein. Complete dissection of the lymph nodes can open the mediastinal space and enable safer dissection of the artery, vein, and bronchi.

The surgical approach differs depending on the completeness of the pulmonary fissure. When the fissure is fused and not well developed, we prefer to perform the steps in the following order (Fig. 9.7): (1) division of the inferior pulmonary ligament, (2) isolation and division of the inferior pulmonary vein, (3) isolation and division of the

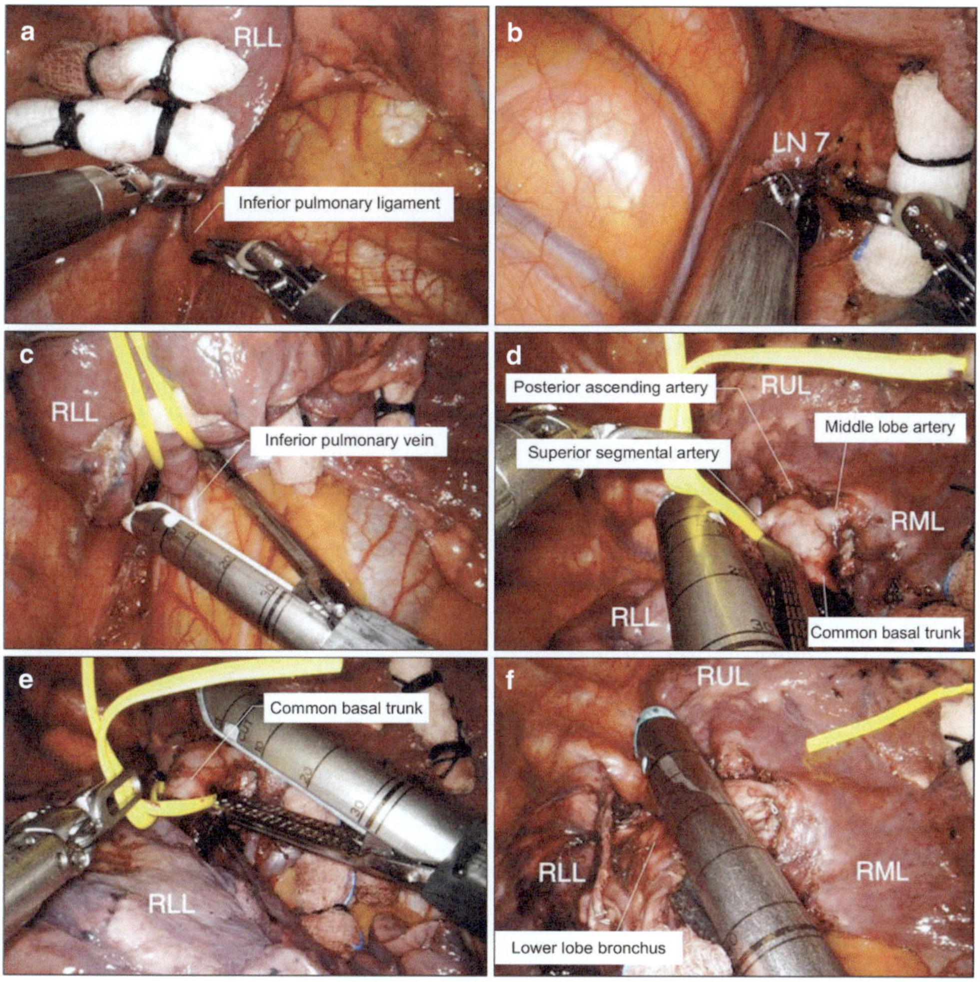

Fig. 9.7 Robotic right lower lobe (RLL) lobectomy. (**a**) Division of the inferior pulmonary ligament. (**b**) Dissection of lymph node (LN) station 7. (**c**) Division of the inferior pulmonary vein. (**d**) Division of the superior segmental artery. (**e**) Division of the common basal trunk. (**f**) Division of the lower lobe bronchus. *RUL* right upper lobe, *RML* right middle lobe

lower lobe artery, and (4) isolation and division of the lower lobe bronchus.

If the fissure is well developed, we prefer a caudal approach, which is described in the section dealing with left lower lobectomy.

Step 1: Division of the Inferior Pulmonary Ligament

The lung is retracted superiorly using Cadiere forceps, and the surgeon begins to divide the inferior edge of the inferior pulmonary ligament using long bipolar forceps. An assistant can help retract the lung superiorly using a long sponge stick. The inferior pulmonary ligament is divided with all surrounding tissues, and lymph node stations 7, 8, and 9 can be removed.

Step 2: Isolation and Division of the Inferior Pulmonary Vein

Next, the lung is retracted anteriorly to expose the subcarinal area using the rolled-up gauze to avoid direct grasping. After dissection of the subcarinal lymph node, the RLL is retracted posteriorly, and the inferior pulmonary vein is carefully dissected. The mediastinal pleura should be completely dissected to identify the middle lobe vein and the right inferior pulmonary vein. The inferior pulmonary vein is encircled with a vessel loop and then divided using a robotic stapler.

Step 3: Isolation and Division of the Lower Lobe Artery

The anterior part of the major fissure between the RLL and the RML is dissected using long bipolar forceps, and the hilar lymph nodes are removed. We prefer to divide the fused major fissure between the RLL and the RML using a robotic stapler to achieve better exposure of the lower lobe artery in the interlobar space. Complete dissection should be continued until the superior segmental and ascending posterior arteries are identified.

Once the superior segmental artery and basal trunk are exposed, they can be divided in 1 step or 2 steps. We prefer a 2-step division, in which the superior segmental artery is divided first with a robotic stapler, and then the basal trunk is divided with a robotic stapler.

Step 4: Isolation and Division of the Lower Lobe Bronchus

After division of the pulmonary artery, all hilar lymph nodes should be removed. The lower lobe bronchus is divided using a robotic stapler. Compromising the middle lobe bronchus should be carefully avoided. Next, the specimen is removed using a specimen bag via the utility incision.

Left Upper Lobectomy

The left upper lobe (LUL) pulmonary branches may arise in a fairly random order, and they frequently form small trunks of two or more branches. Some branches are too small and short to place the stapler. Therefore, careful dissection of the vessel and placement of the stapler must be performed to avoid vessel laceration. Some branches of the pulmonary artery are too small and short, and they can be ligated with robotic Hem-o-Lok clips.

Although the sequence of steps in dissection may vary to some degree due to variations in anatomy, we prefer to perform the steps in the following order (Fig. 9.8): (1) isolation and division of the superior pulmonary vein, (2) division of the lingular segmental arteries and posterior pulmonary artery branches, (3) isolation and division of the LUL bronchus, and (4) isolation and division of the apicoposterior segmental artery.

Step 1: Isolation and Division of the Superior Pulmonary Vein

The lung is retraced posteriorly to expose the hilum, and the anterior mediastinal pleura is opened. Dissection should be continued until the bifurcation between the superior pulmonary vein and the inferior pulmonary vein is identified. The division of the left superior pulmonary vein is easier than that of the RUL vein due to the absence of the RML vein. The superior pulmonary vein is encircled with a vessel loop, and then divided using a robotic stapler.

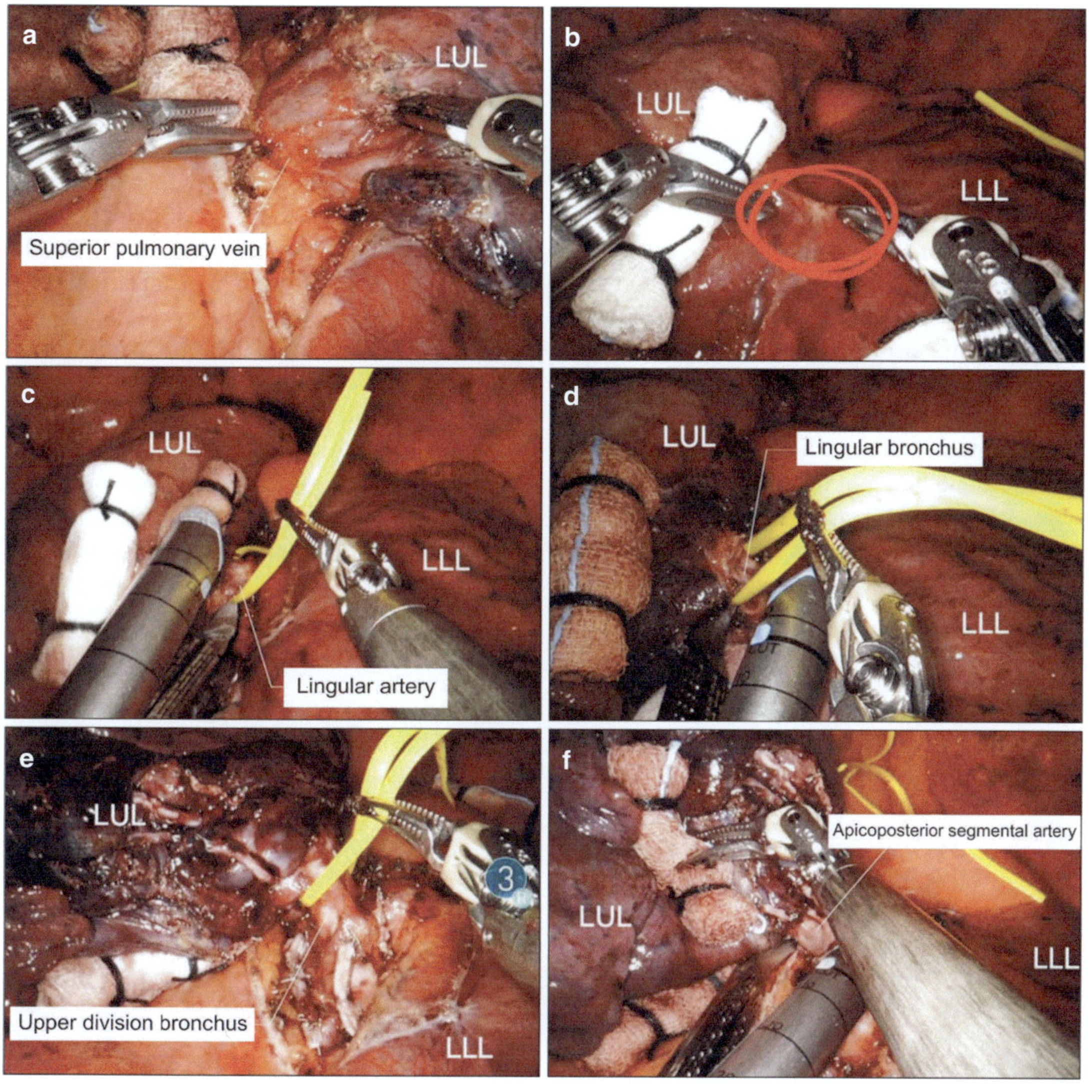

Fig. 9.8 Robotic left upper lobectomy. (**a**) Isolation of the superior pulmonary vein. (**b**) Dissection of the fissure. (**c**) Division of the lingular segmental artery. (**d**) Division of the lingular bronchus. (**e**) Division of the upper division bronchus. (**f**) Division of the apicoposterior segmental artery. *LUL* left upper lobe, *LLL* left lower lobe

Step 2: Division of the Lingular Segmental Arteries and Posterior Pulmonary Artery Branches

Next, we dissect the fissure using long bipolar forceps. Retraction of the lung by the robotic wrist with rolled-up gauze facilitates dissection of the fissure. After the fissure dissection, the anatomy of the pulmonary artery is identified. Once the superior segmental artery is identified, a tunnel for fissure division can be created. The fused anterior part of the major fissure can be divided using a robotic stapler through the tunnel. The nodal tissues are dissected to facilitate the subsequent passage of the robotic stapler. Once the entire interlobar artery is clearly exposed, the posterior pulmonary artery branches and lingular segmental artery are identified along the upper edge of the interlobar artery. The posterior pulmonary artery branches and lingular segmental artery are encircled with a vessel loop and divided using a robotic stapler in order. If the pulmonary artery branch is too small and short for a stapler, the robotic Hem-o-Lok clips can be used to ligate it.

Step 3: Isolation and Division of the LUL Bronchus

The upper lobar bronchus is located in the middle of the major fissure, and it is usually exposed after division of the lingular segmental arteries and posterior pulmonary artery branches. The lung is retracted anteriorly and the nodal tissues are removed. The normal LUL bronchus is divided into the upper division bronchus and the lingular bronchus, and they can be divided in 1 step or 2 steps. We prefer a 2-step division, in which the lingular bronchus and the upper division bronchus are divided using a robotic stapler in order.

Step 4: Isolation and Division of the Apicoposterior Segmental Artery

The apicoposterior segmental artery arises from the posterosuperior aspect of the left pulmonary artery and passes through the front of the LUL bronchus. The apicoposterior segmental artery is clearly exposed after division of the LUL bronchus. The apicoposterior segmental artery and remaining posterior pulmonary artery branches are isolated and divided using a robotic stapler in order. When the posterior pulmonary artery branches are multiple and small, they can be ligated using robotic Hem-o-Lok clips. Next, the specimen is removed using a specimen bag via the utility incision.

Left Lower Lobectomy

Left lower robotic lobectomy is performed in a manner similar to that of right lower lobectomy. When the fissure is well developed, we prefer a caudal approach (Fig. 9.9): (1) division of the inferior pulmonary ligament, (2) isolation and division of the inferior pulmonary vein, (3) isolation and division of the lower lobe bronchus, and (4) isolation and division of the inferior pulmonary artery. If the fissure is fused and not well developed, we prefer the order described in the section describing right lower lobectomy.

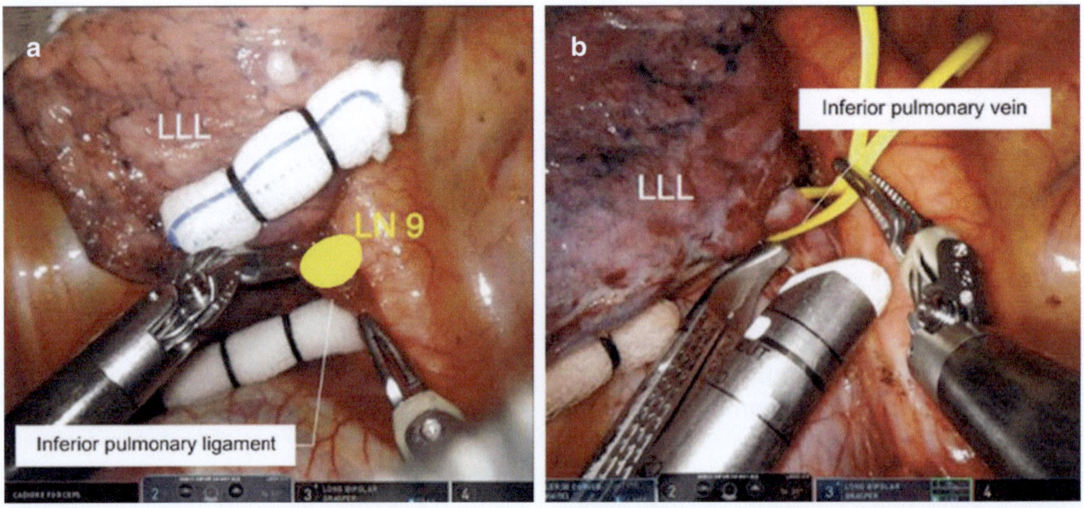

Fig. 9.9 Robotic left lower lobectomy. (**a**) Division of the inferior pulmonary ligament. (**b**) Division of the inferior pulmonary vein. (**c**) Identification of the anatomy of the pulmonary artery. (**d**) Division of the superior segmental bronchus. (**e**) Division of the superior segmental artery. (**f**) Division of the common basal trunk. *LUL* left upper lobe, *LLL* left lower lobe, *LN* lymph node

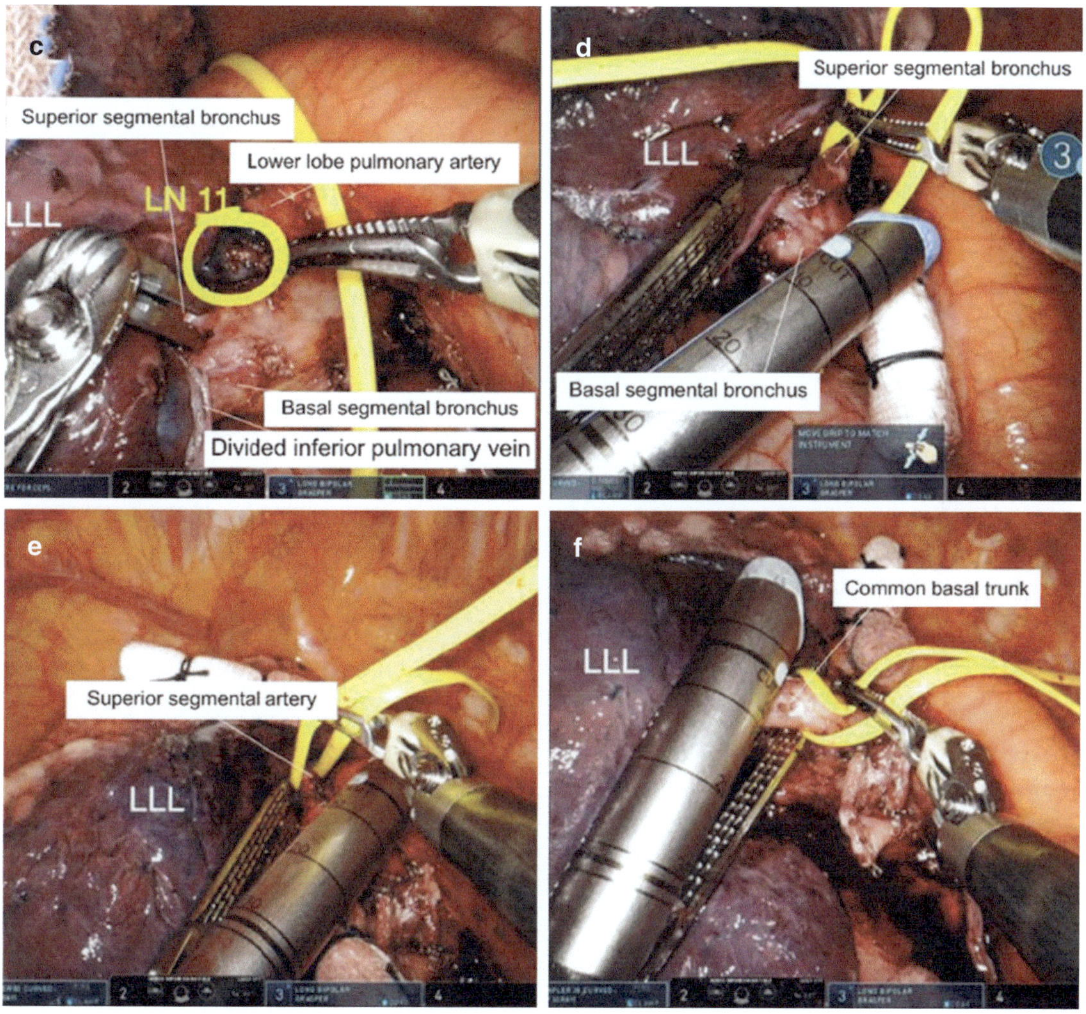

Fig. 9.9 (continued)

Step 1: Division of the Inferior Pulmonary Ligament

The lung is retracted superiorly using Cadiere forceps and the surgeon begins to divide the inferior edge of the inferior pulmonary ligament using long bipolar forceps. An assistant can provide superior traction of the lung using a long sponge stick. The inferior pulmonary ligament is divided with all surrounding tissues, and lymph node stations 7, 8, and 9 can be removed.

Step 2: Isolation and Division of the Inferior Pulmonary Vein

Once the inferior pulmonary vein is exposed, the hilum is dissected anteriorly to identify the anatomy of the pulmonary vein. The bifurcation of the inferior pulmonary vein and superior pulmonary vein should be exposed and identified. The inferior pulmonary vein is encircled with a vessel loop, and then divided using a robotic stapler.

Step 3: Isolation and Division of the Lower Lobe Bronchus

The lung is retracted anteriorly, and the left lower bronchus is dissected. The left lower bronchus divides into a superior segmental bronchus and four basal segmental bronchi. All hilar lymph nodes are removed, and the superior segmental bronchus is identified. Completion of the fissure can be performed using a robotic stapler, which facilitates visualization of the bronchus and artery. The left lower bronchus can be divided by 1 step or 2 steps, and we prefer a 2-step division. The superior segmental bronchus and basal segmental bronchus can be divided using a robotic stapler in order.

Step 4: Isolation and Division of the Lower Lobe Pulmonary Artery

After division of the left lower bronchus, the fissure is dissected to identify the anatomy of the pulmonary artery. The left lower pulmonary artery divides into the superior segmental artery and the common basal trunk. Once the superior segment and basal trunk are exposed, they can be divided in 1 step or 2 steps. We prefer a 2-step division, wherein these structures are divided using a robotic stapler in order. Next, the remainder of the fissure is divided using a robotic stapler. Subsequently, the specimen is removed using a specimen bag via the utility incision.

9.5 Conclusion

Herein, we have presented a review of robotic lobectomy, focusing on several key technical points for a successful operation. Robotic lobectomy is feasible and safe, and it may be useful for more challenging surgical procedures. Although the learning curve for robotic lobectomy is steep, the technology of robotic surgical systems is still evolving, and upgraded systems will enhance the speed, accuracy, and safety of robotic lobectomy in the future.

Conflict of Interest No potential conflict of interest relevant to this article was reported.

References

1. Yang CF, Sun Z, Speicher PJ, et al. Use and outcomes of minimally invasive lobectomy for stage I non-small cell lung cancer in the National Cancer Data Base. Ann Thorac Surg. 2016;101:1037–42.
2. Emmert A, Straube C, Buentzel J, Roever C. Robotic versus thoracoscopic lung resection: a systematic review and meta-analysis. Medicine (Baltimore). 2017;96:e7633.
3. O'Sullivan KE, Kreaden US, Hebert AE, Eaton D, Redmond KC. A systematic review and meta-analysis of robotic versus open and video-assisted thoracoscopic surgery approaches for lobectomy. Interact Cardiovasc Thorac Surg. 2019;28:526–34.
4. Linsky P, Wei B. Robotic lobectomy. J Visc Surg. 2017;3:132.
5. Kneuertz PJ, D'Souza DM, Richardson M, Abdel-Rasoul M, Moffatt-Bruce SD, Merritt RE. Long-term oncologic outcomes after robotic lobectomy for early-stage non-small-cell lung cancer versus video-assisted thoracoscopic and open thoracotomy approach. Clin Lung Cancer. 2020;21:214–24.
6. Roviaro G, Rebuffat C, Varoli F, Vergani C, Mariani C, Maciocco M. Videoendoscopic pulmonary lobectomy for cancer. Surg Laparosc Endosc. 1992;2:244–7.
7. Berfield KS, Farjah F, Mulligan MS. Video-assisted thoracoscopic lobectomy for lung cancer. Ann Thorac Surg. 2019;107:603–9.
8. McKenna RJ Jr. Lobectomy by video-assisted thoracic surgery with mediastinal node sampling for lung cancer. J Thorac Cardiovasc Surg. 1994;107:879–82.
9. Landreneau RJ, Mack MJ, Hazelrigg SR, et al. Video-assisted thoracic surgery: basic technical concepts and intercostal approach strategies. Ann Thorac Surg. 1992;54:800–7.
10. Lin J. Robotic lobectomy: revolution or evolution? J Thorac Dis. 2017;9:2876–80.
11. Park BJ, Flores RM, Rusch VW. Robotic assistance for video-assisted thoracic surgical lobectomy: technique and initial results. J Thorac Cardiovasc Surg. 2006;131:54–9.
12. Ricciardi S, Cardillo G, Zirafa CC, Davini F, Melfi F. Robotic lobectomies: when and why? J Visc Surg. 2017;3:112.
13. Melfi FM, Menconi GF, Mariani AM, Angeletti CA. Early experience with robotic technology for thoracoscopic surgery. Eur J Cardiothorac Surg. 2002;21:864–8.
14. Zirafa CC, Romano G, Key TH, Davini F, Melfi F. The evolution of robotic thoracic surgery. Ann Cardiothorac Surg. 2019;8:210–7.
15. Galetta D, Casiraghi M, Pardolesi A, Borri A, Spaggiari L. New stapling devices in robotic surgery. J Visc Surg. 2017;3:45.
16. Farivar AS, Cerfolio RJ, Vallieres E, et al. Comparing robotic lung resection with thoracotomy and video-assisted thoracoscopic surgery cases entered into the

Society of Thoracic Surgeons database. Innovations (Phila). 2014;9:10–5.

17. Kent M, Wang T, Whyte R, Curran T, Flores R, Gangadharan S. Open, video-assisted thoracic surgery, and robotic lobectomy: review of a national database. Ann Thorac Surg. 2014;97:236–44.
18. Veronesi G, Galetta D, Maisonneuve P, et al. Four-arm robotic lobectomy for the treatment of early-stage lung cancer. J Thorac Cardiovasc Surg. 2010;140:19–25.
19. Adams RD, Bolton WD, Stephenson JE, Henry G, Robbins ET, Sommers E. Initial multicenter community robotic lobectomy experience: comparisons to a national database. Ann Thorac Surg. 2014;97:1893–900.
20. Bao F, Zhang C, Yang Y, He Z, Wang L, Hu J. Comparison of robotic and video-assisted thoracic surgery for lung cancer: a propensity-matched analysis. J Thorac Dis. 2016;8:1798–803.
21. Yang HX. Long-term survival of early-stage non-small cell lung cancer patients who underwent robotic procedure: a propensity score-matched study. Chin J Cancer. 2016;35:66.
22. Qiu T, Zhao Y, Xuan Y, Jiao W. Robotic-assisted double-sleeve lobectomy. J Thorac Dis. 2017;9:E21–5.
23. Wilson JL, Louie BE, Cerfolio RJ, et al. The prevalence of nodal upstaging during robotic lung resection in early stage non-small cell lung cancer. Ann Thorac Surg. 2014;97:1901–7.
24. Casiraghi M, Spaggiari L. Robotic lobectomy has the greatest benefit in patients with marginal pulmonary function. J Thorac Dis. 2019;11(Suppl 3):S322–4.
25. Veronesi G, Novellis P, Difrancesco O, Dylewski M. Robotic assisted lobectomy for locally advanced lung cancer. J Visc Surg. 2017;3:78.
26. Wei B, Cerfolio RJ. Robotic lobectomy and segmentectomy: technical details and results. Surg Clin N Am. 2017;97:771–82.
27. Melfi FM, Mussi A. Robotically assisted lobectomy: learning curve and complications. Thorac Surg Clin. 2008;18:289–95.
28. Gharagozloo F, Margolis M, Tempesta B, Strother E, Najam F. Robot-assisted lobectomy for early-stage lung cancer: report of 100 consecutive cases. Ann Thorac Surg. 2009;88:380–4.
29. Arnold BN, Thomas DC, Bhatnagar V, et al. Defining the learning curve in robot-assisted thoracoscopic lobectomy. Surgery. 2019;165:450–4.
30. Song G, Sun X, Miao S, et al. Learning curve for robot-assisted lobectomy of lung cancer. J Thorac Dis. 2019;11:2431–7.
31. Jang HJ, Lee HS, Park SY, Zo JI. Comparison of the early robot-assisted lobectomy experience to video-assisted thoracic surgery lobectomy for lung cancer: a single-institution case series matching study. Innovations (Phila). 2011;6:305–10.
32. Pearlstein DP. Robotic lobectomy utilizing the robotic stapler. Ann Thorac Surg. 2016;102:e591–3.
33. Pardolesi A, Bertolaccini L, Brandolini J, Solli P, Novellis P, Veronesi G. Four arms robotic-assisted pulmonary resection-left upper lobectomy: how to do it. J Visc Surg. 2018;4:109.
34. Cerfolio RJ, Bryant AS, Skylizard L, Minnich DJ. Initial consecutive experience of completely portal robotic pulmonary resection with 4 arms. J Thorac Cardiovasc Surg. 2011;142:740–6.

Part II

Esophagus

Thoracoscopic Esophagectomy for Esophageal Cancer: Detailed Procedures and Review

10

Seong Yong Park

Abstract

Thoracoscopic esophagectomy for esophageal cancer can be performed in multiple positions, such as the lateral decubitus position or prone position, using various techniques. Each approach has its own advantages and disadvantages, and surgeons can select an appropriate approach based on their preferences. Except for the reduction of pulmonary complications, the benefits of thoracoscopic esophagectomy, including oncologic outcomes, have not been proven scientifically. This review describes the approaches and procedures of thoracoscopic esophagectomy and presents scientific evidence for this procedure.

Keywords

Esophageal cancer · Thoracoscopy

10.1 Introduction

Despite advances in perioperative management, esophagectomy for esophageal cancer remains one of the most invasive gastrointestinal surgical procedures, with serious postoperative complications [1]. The morbidity and mortality rates have been reported to be up to 60% and 3.4%, respectively, according to a large Japanese national report [2]. Therefore, esophagectomy via the thoracoscopic and/or laparoscopic approach can be a very attractive and less invasive alternative to conventional open esophagectomy for reducing postoperative morbidity and mortality. This increase in the popularity of thoracoscopic esophagectomy might also be related to technical advances in thoracoscopic equipment such as dissectors, laparoscopic coagulating shears, and vessel-sealing systems, which are now available for thoracoscopic esophageal resection and extended mediastinal lymphadenectomy [1]. Historically, thoracoscopic esophagectomy was first introduced in 1992 by Cuschieri et al. [3], in a report presenting a series of five patients who underwent thoracoscopic surgery combined with laparotomy. DePaula et al. [4] reported their experience of laparoscopic transhiatal esophagectomy in 1995 and Luketich et al. [5] reported acceptable outcomes from 222 patients who underwent a combined thoracoscopic and laparoscopic approach for esophageal cancer in 2003. In recent years, various approaches for thoracoscopic esophagectomy have been attempted.

S. Y. Park (✉)
Department of Thoracic and Cardiovascular Surgery, Samsung Medical Center, Sungkyunkwan University School of Medicine, Seoul, Republic of Korea

K. Kim et al. (eds.), *Techniques in Minimally Invasive Thoracic Surgery*,
https://doi.org/10.1007/978-981-19-2472-9_10

10.2 Various Approaches of Thoracoscopic Esophagectomy

Thoracoscopic esophagectomy can be performed with the patient in the lateral decubitus position. It can offer a similar view to traditional thoracotomy, with the advantage that urgent thoracotomy conversion can be performed easily. However, this position requires total lung collapse with 1-lung ventilation, which is frequently associated with pulmonary complications. To overcome the issues related to 1-lung ventilation, thoracoscopic esophagectomy in the prone position has also been attempted. Palanivelu et al. [6] reported that thoracoscopic transthoracic esophagectomy in the prone position in 130 patients was technically feasible, with a low respiratory complication rate and a shorter operative time due to the excellent exposure of the operative field and better ergonomics. However, it is difficult to perform urgent conversion to traditional thoracotomy. In addition, dissection of the left recurrent laryngeal nerve (RLN) lymph nodes, where metastasis most frequently develops in esophageal squamous cell carcinoma, is technically challenging in the prone position. To overcome the abovementioned problem while maintaining the benefits of the prone position, thoracoscopic esophagectomy in the semi-prone position has recently become popular among surgeons [7].

Surgeons have also attempted transhiatal and transcervical esophagectomy. Transhiatal open esophagectomy was first reported by Orringer and Sloan [8] and is regarded as less invasive and radical than transthoracic open esophagectomy. This procedure can be modified with laparoscopy and can be considered a minimally invasive esophagectomy. Although the transhiatal approach is regarded as less invasive than the transthoracic approach, mediastinal lymph node dissection is insufficient for the treatment of esophageal cancer. Therefore, the video-assisted transcervical approach for the dissection of the proximal and mid-esophagus has been implemented in combination with a transhiatal approach to improve the quality of mediastinal lymph node dissection without transthoracic dissection and 1-lung ventilation at some Japanese institutions [9]. This procedure is not popular in Korea.

10.3 Personal Procedures Performed by the Author

The author prefers McKeown 3-field esophagectomy with cervical anastomosis using thoracoscopy. This section describes the author's personal procedures of thoracoscopic esophagectomy in the lateral decubitus position. The patient is placed in the left lateral decubitus position after double-lumen intubation. A 4-cm working window is made first at the fourth intercostal space anterior axillary line to confirm pleural adhesion. After the absence of pleural adhesion is confirmed, CO_2 (20 mmHg) was used for lung collapse. After sufficient lung collapse with CO_2 insufflation, the full size of the working window and other trocars are inserted at the sixth intercostal space of the scapular tip and the seventh (or eighth) intercostal space, as shown in Fig. 10.1. The author personally prefers a working window because a thick instrument such as a tracheal retractor can be inserted through a working window.

The sequence of the procedures is described in Fig. 10.2. The dissection is initiated at the azygos arch; the mediastinal pleura over the azygos vein is opened, and the azygos vein is stapled with an endoscopic vascular stapler. The right bronchial artery, which arises from the intercostal artery, can be detected below the azygous vein, and the right bronchial artery is usually sacrificed with a metal clip (Fig. 10.3a). At this level, the thoracic duct can be found between the azygous vein and aorta, with the dissection plane just outside of the thoracic duct for en bloc resection of the thoracic duct (Fig. 10.3b). The dissection of the dorsal side of the upper esophagus continued from the upper mediastinum to the thoracic inlet (Fig. 10.4a). For the blunt dissection of this rea, any energy device such as a harmonic scalpel is

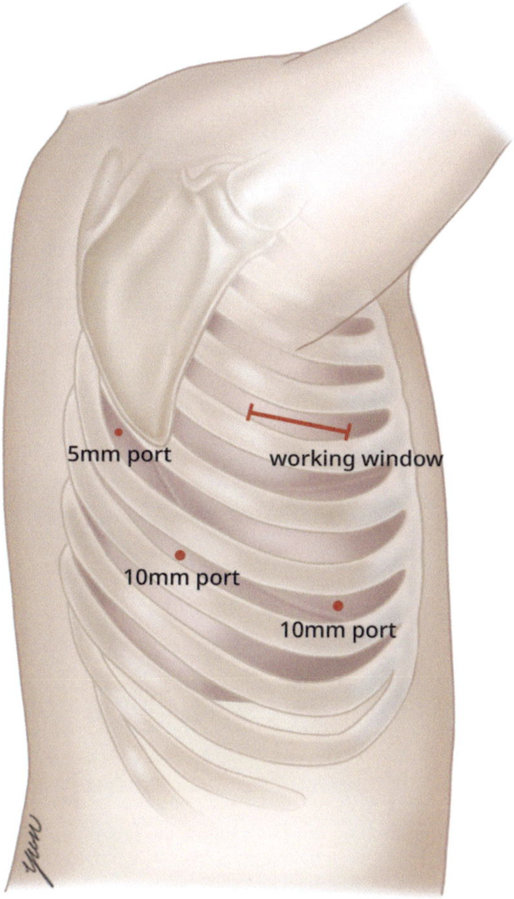

Fig. 10.1 The position and placement of the trocars in thoracoscopic esophagectomy with the patient in the lateral decubitus position. A 4-cm-long working window is made at the fourth intercostal space, a 5-mm port is placed at the sixth intercostal space and scapular tip, and two 10-mm ports are placed at the seventh or eighth intercostal space

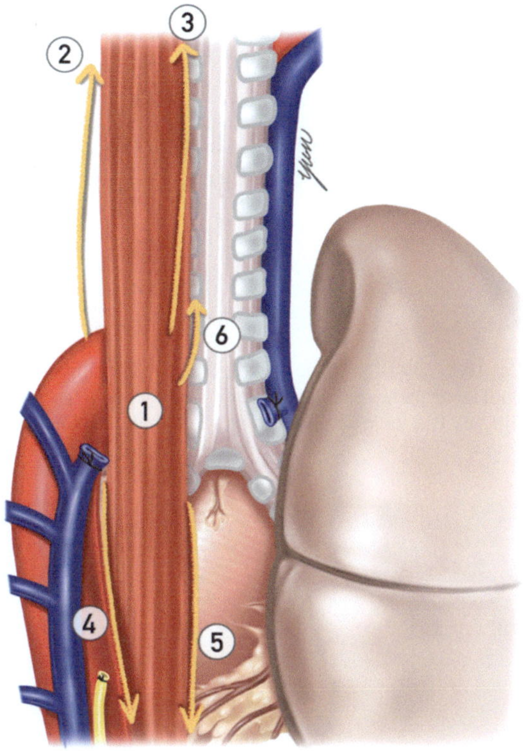

Fig. 10.2 The sequence of thoracoscopic esophagectomy. (*1*) division of the azygos vein; (*2*) dissection of the dorsal side of the upper esophagus; (*3*) dissection of the right recurrent laryngeal nerve lymph nodes; (*4*) dissection of the dorsal side of the lower esophagus; (*5*) dissection of the subcarinal lymph nodes and the ventral side of the esophagus; (*6*) dissection of the left recurrent laryngeal nerve lymph nodes

usually used. After dissection to the thoracic inlet, the mediastinal pleura over the vagus nerve is opened from the azygous vein level to the edge of the right subclavian artery. At this level, the right RLN lymph nodes are carefully dissected after finding and preserving the right RLN. The RLN is identified at the caudal end of the right subclavian artery. Lymph nodes around the nerve are dissected and resected up to the cervical level with meticulous care to prevent nerve injury (Fig. 10.4b). The sharp dissection around the nerve is usually done with long Metzenbaum scissors to prevent thermal injury. Next, the anterior part of the upper esophagus is dissected from the trachea.

After dissection of the upper esophagus, dissection between the vertebral body and esophagus is performed on the diaphragm side. The thoracic duct is attached to the specimen side (esophagus) for en bloc resection. At the diaphragm level, the thoracic duct is ligated to the metal clip to prevent chylothorax (Fig. 10.5a). Dissection of the lower esophagus is performed, with the contralateral mediastinal pleura (left side mediastinal pleura) usually saved in cT1 or T2 lesions (Fig. 10.5b). In the case of a T3 lesion at the lower esophagus, the left side mediastinal pleura is also dissected en bloc. Then, dissection

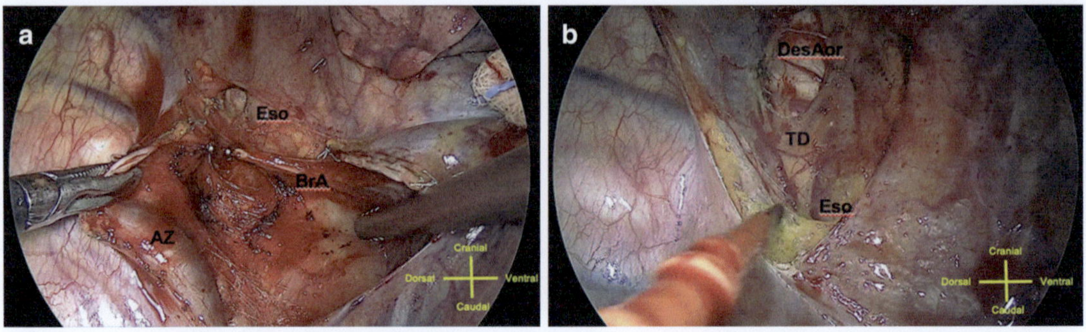

Fig. 10.3 Division of the azygos vein. (**a**) The right bronchial artery below the azygos vein is divided with a metal clip. (**b**) The thoracic duct can be found between the azygous vein and aorta. *AZ* azygos vein, *BrA* right bronchial artery, *Eso* esophagus, *TD* thoracic duct, *DesAor* descending thoracic aorta

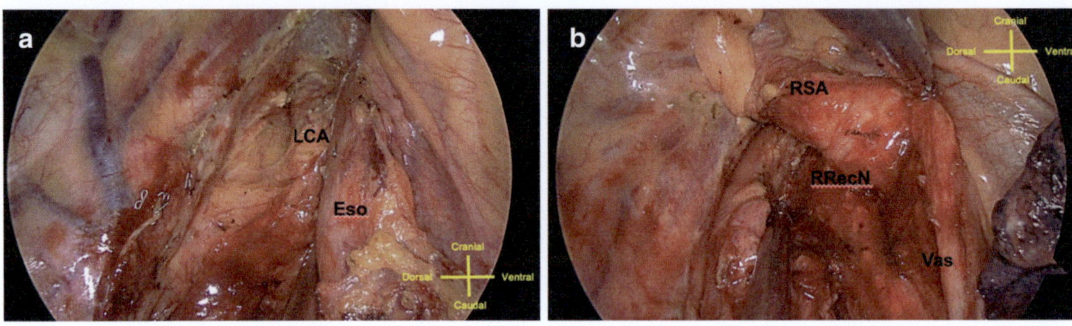

Fig. 10.4 Dissection of the upper esophagus. (**a**) Dissection of the dorsal side of the upper esophagus to the thoracic inlet. (**b**) Dissection of the right recurrent laryngeal nerve lymph nodes. *Eso* esophagus, *LAC* left carotid artery, *RSA* right subclavian artery, *Vas* vagus nerve, *RRecN* right recurrent laryngeal nerve

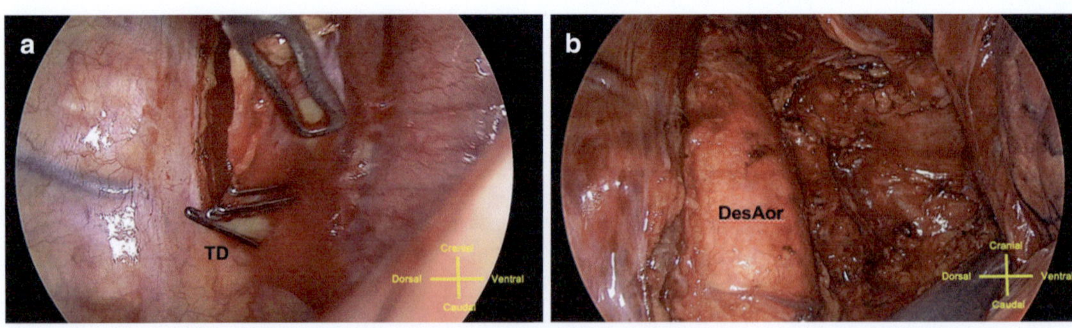

Fig. 10.5 Dissection of the lower esophagus. (**a**) Ligation of the thoracic duct at the diaphragm level. (**b**) Dissection of the lower esophagus with denudation of the descending thoracic aorta. *TD* thoracic duct, *DesAor* descending thoracic aorta

of the subcarinal lymph nodes begins. The pulmonary branches of the vagus nerve, which runs along the right main bronchus, are preserved, and the vagus nerve is cut just below the pulmonary branches of the right vagus nerve (Fig. 10.6a). With the retraction of the pulmonary branches to the cranial side, the subcarinal lymph nodes are dissected from the main bronchus with an en bloc attachment to the esophagus (Fig. 10.6b). At this phase, the dissection must be performed carefully

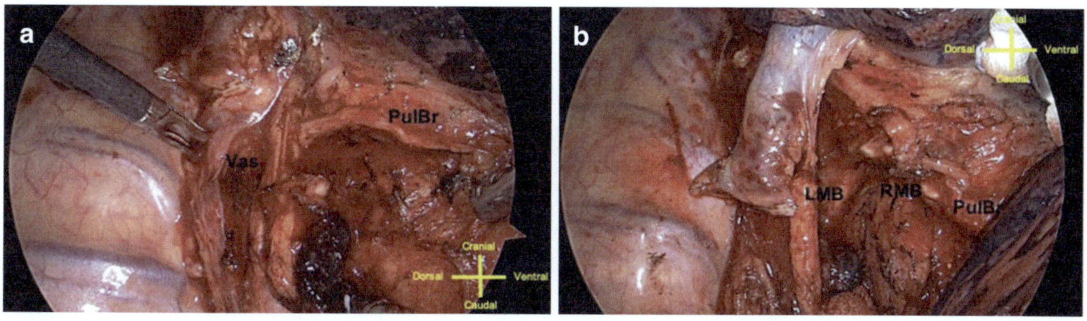

Fig. 10.6 Dissection of subcarinal lymph nodes. (**a**) Saving the right pulmonary branches of the vagus nerve during subcarinal lymph node dissection. (**b**) The subcarinal lymph nodes are dissected while attached to the esophagus, in an en bloc manner. *Vas* vagus nerve, *PulBr* right pulmonary branch of the vagus nerve, *RMB* right main bronchus, *LMB* left main bronchus

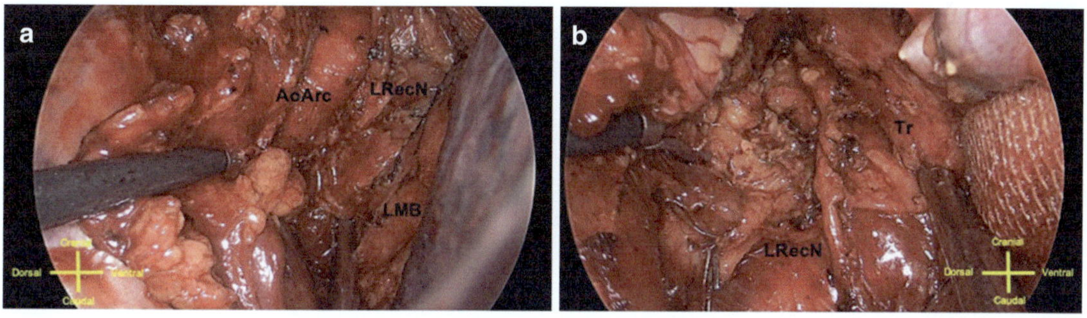

Fig. 10.7 Dissection of the left recurrent laryngeal area. (**a**) Dissection of the left tracheobronchial lymph nodes. (**b**) Dissection of the left recurrent laryngeal nerve lymph nodes. *AoArc* aortic arch, *LMB* left main bronchus, *LRecN* left recurrent laryngeal nerve, *Tr* trachea

to avoid injury to the left main bronchus and inferior pulmonary vein. After the dissection of the subcarinal lymph nodes, the dissection continues to the diaphragm side, and the right crus muscle can be found during the thoracic phase.

The esophagus is then lifted upward and dissection around the left side of the esophagus is performed to identify the left RLN. These dissections usually begin just above the left main bronchus, with the left RLN, which encircles the aortic arch, found easily at this level. The left pulmonary artery is exposed to dissect the left tracheobronchial lymph nodes between the aortic arch and the left main bronchus (Fig. 10.7a). The tissues between the esophagus and trachea are dissected and the trachea is retracted anteriorly by an assistant using a tracheal retractor. The soft tissues and lymph nodes around the left RLN are carefully dissected from the aortic arch to the cervical level (Fig. 10.7b). Thus, esophageal mobilization and mediastinal lymphadenectomy are completed.

Abdominal procedures are performed through an upper midline abdominal incision, giving access to the greater omentum, short gastric vessels, and lesser omentum, while avoiding injury to the right gastroepiploic and right gastric vessels. The fat tissue over the left gastric artery is dissected, the artery is divided, and the paracardial, left gastric, and celiac lymph nodes are dissected. Then, bilateral neck dissection is performed via a collar incision, and an anastomosis is made at the neck. The gastric conduit is pulled up to the neck through the posterior mediastinal or substernal route. The cervical esophagus and gastric conduit are then anastomosed using a hand-sewn maneuver. The anastomosis can also be performed at the thoracic inlet, similar to the Ivor–Lewis operation; the methods of anastomosis will be described in other papers.

10.4 Surgical Pitfalls

During left RLN lymph node dissection, the trachea must be retracted gently. Rough retraction can result in catastrophic events, such as tracheal injury. In addition, the esophagus must be lifted upward carefully to avoid traction injury of the left RLN. Dissection must also be performed carefully around the left main bronchus. The left inferior pulmonary vein is located at the end of the left main bronchus, which can be injured during dissection. Some surgeons believe that saving the right bronchial artery is important for preventing pulmonary complications, but the author's routine practice is ligation of the right bronchial artery for better exposure of the left RLN area. Sacrificing the right bronchial artery did not seem to increase pulmonary complications.

10.5 Literature Review

Despite the increased popularity of thoracoscopic esophagectomy, scientific evidence for this procedure is unclear. The short-term and long-term outcomes of thoracoscopic esophagectomy in retrospective studies are summarized in Table 10.1. In many studies, the operative time was found to be longer in thoracoscopic esophagectomy than in open esophagectomy [2, 10–12]. However, in terms of blood loss, hospital stay, and pulmonary complications, several papers reported better outcomes for thoracoscopic esophagectomy. Tapias et al. [13] also reported that thoracoscopic esophagectomy could be done safely even after neoadjuvant therapy. Regarding overall survival, several retrospective studies showed better overall survival in patients who underwent thoracoscopic esophagectomy [10, 14], but the results must be interpreted cautiously because of possible confounding factors or selection bias. A recent meta-analysis found comparable long-term survival rates between thoracoscopic esophagectomy and conventional open esophagectomy [15]. However, as no randomized controlled trials have been performed to compare the long-term survival of patients undergoing thoracoscopic esophagectomy and open esophagectomy, the benefits of thoracoscopic esophagectomy for oncologic patients have not been scientifically shown, especially in patients with esophageal squamous cell carcinoma.

Nationwide studies and prospective studies have also reported data on the short-term outcomes of thoracoscopic esophagectomy (Table 10.2). Interestingly, the incidence of pulmonary complications seems to be lower after thoracoscopic esophagectomy, whereas overall surgical complications are more common after esophagectomy; anastomotic leakage [16], intra-abdominal abscess [16], reintervention [16, 17], reoperation [17, 18], and RLN palsy [18] were reported more frequently in thoracoscopic esophagectomy than in open esophagectomy. However, operative mortality was similar between the two surgical methods. The TIME trial, which was a phase III randomized controlled trial that compared thoracoscopic esophagectomy to open esophagectomy, also reported that the incidence of pulmonary infection was considerably lower in the thoracoscopic esophagectomy group than in the open esophagectomy group, and the other complications were comparable between the two groups [19]. Based on the results from previous retrospective, nationwide, and prospective studies, thoracoscopic esophagectomy has been shown to reduce the occurrence of postoperative respiratory complications, whereas other complications are comparable or slightly increased. Therefore, the 2017 esophageal cancer practice guidelines published by the Japan Esophageal Society do not strongly recommend thoracoscopic esophagectomy.

Table 10.1 Comparison of the short-term outcomes between thoracoscopic and open esophagectomy in retrospective series

Author (year)	No. of cases	Operation time (min)	Blood loss (mL)	Mortality (%)	Hospital stay (day)	Pulmonary complication (%)	Anastomotic leakage (%)	Vocal cord palsy (%)	No. of dissected LNs	OS (year)
Osugi et al. (2003) [11]	TE (77) vs. OE (72)	227 vs. 186[a]	284 vs. 310	0 vs. 0	–	15.6 vs. 19.4	1.3 vs. 2.8	14.3 vs. 19.4	33.9 vs. 32.8	55 vs. 57 (5-year OS)
Daiko and Nishimura (2012) [12]	TE (29) vs. OE (30)	322 vs. 335[a]	527 vs. 435	0 vs. 0	20 vs. 20	3 vs. 3	14 vs. 10	17 vs. 20	–	–
Miyasaka et al. (2013) [14]	TE (68) vs. OE (30)	483 vs. 508	364 vs. 975[a]	2.9 vs. 13.3	35.0 vs. 85.5[a]	32.4 vs. 43.3	7.4 vs. 16.7	25 vs. 30	37 vs. 41.5	61.5 vs. 26.7 (5-year OS)[a]
Hsu et al. (2014) [10]	TE (66) vs. OE (63)	511 vs. 461[a]	462 vs. 615	7.6 vs. 7.9	–	10.6 vs. 25.4[a]	27.3 vs. 30.3	–	28.3 vs. 25.7	70.9 vs. 47.6[a]
Takeuchi et al. (2014) [2]	TE (1751) vs. OE (3603)	523 vs. 450[a]	466 vs. 618[a]	3 vs. 3.6	–	15.0 vs. 15.5	14.9 vs. 12.5[a]	–	–	–
Tapias et al. (2016) [13]	TE (56) vs. OE (74)	337.4 vs. 361.6	200 vs. 250[a]	0 vs. 2.7	7 vs. 9[a]	8.9 vs. 29.7[a]	0 vs. 1.4	0 vs. 4	20 vs 20	49.6 vs. 60.9

LN laryngeal nerve, *TE* thoracoscopic esophagectomy, *OE* open esophagectomy, *OS* overall survival
[a] Statistically significant

Table 10.2 Comparison of the short-term outcomes between thoracoscopic esophagectomy and open esophagectomy in nationwide or prospective data

Author (year)	Country	Study design	Period	No. of cases (OE vs. TE)	Respiratory complications (OE vs. TE)	Surgical complications (OE vs. TE)	30-Day mortality (OE vs. TE)
Biere et al. (2012) [19]	Europe	Randomized controlled trial	2005–2008	56 vs. 59	29% vs. 9%, $p = 0.008$	Equivalent except for pulmonary complications	0% vs. 2%, $p = 0.580$
Seesing et al. (2017) [16]	Netherlands	National data (propensity score matching)	2011–2015	433 vs. 433	34.2% vs. 35.8%, $p = 0.669$	More frequent anastomotic leakage, intra-abdominal abscess, and reintervention in TE	3% vs. 4.9%, $p = 0.209$
Mamidanna et al. (2012) [17]	England	National data (population-based study)	2005–2010	6347 vs. 1155	Equivalent	More frequent reoperation and reintervention in TE	4.8% vs. 4.2%, $p = 0.605$
Takeuchi et al. (2017) [18]	Japan	National data	2011–2012	3515 vs. 3515	5.1% vs. 3.6%, $p = 0.002$	More frequent reoperation (5.3% vs. 7%) and recurrent laryngeal nerve palsy (8.1% vs. 10.3%) in TE	0.9% vs. 1.1%

OE open esophagectomy, *TE* thoracoscopic esophagectomy

10.6 Conclusion

Thoracoscopic esophagectomy for esophageal cancer can be performed in various positions, such as the lateral decubitus position or prone position, using various techniques. Each approach has advantages and disadvantages, and surgeons can select an appropriate approach based on their preferences. Thoracoscopic esophagectomy in the lateral decubitus position offers a familiar anatomical view similar to that of conventional open thoracotomy. The benefits of thoracoscopic esophagectomy, including oncologic outcomes, have not been proven scientifically, except for the reduction of pulmonary complications.

Conflict of Interest No potential conflict of interest relevant to this article was reported.

References

1. Booka E, Takeuchi H, Nishi T, et al. The impact of postoperative complications on survivals after esophagectomy for esophageal cancer. Medicine (Baltimore). 2015;94:e1369.
2. Takeuchi H, Miyata H, Gotoh M, et al. A risk model for esophagectomy using data of 5354 patients included in a Japanese nationwide web-based database. Ann Surg. 2014;260:259–66.
3. Cuschieri A, Shimi S, Banting S. Endoscopic oesophagectomy through a right thoracoscopic approach. J R Coll Surg Edinb. 1992;37:7–11.
4. DePaula AL, Hashiba K, Ferreira EA, de Paula RA, Grecco E. Laparoscopic transhiatal esophagectomy with esophagogastroplasty. Surg Laparosc Endosc. 1995;5:1–5.
5. Luketich JD, Alvelo-Rivera M, Buenaventura PO, et al. Minimally invasive esophagectomy: outcomes in 222 patients. Ann Surg. 2003;238:486–94.
6. Palanivelu C, Prakash A, Senthilkumar R, et al. Minimally invasive esophagectomy: thoracoscopic mobilization of the esophagus and mediastinal lymphadenectomy in prone position: experience of 130 patients. J Am Coll Surg. 2006;203:7–16.
7. Seesing MF, Goense L, Ruurda JP, Luyer MD, Nieuwenhuijzen GA, van Hillegersberg R. Minimally invasive esophagectomy: a propensity score-matched analysis of semiprone versus prone position. Surg Endosc. 2018;32:2758–65.
8. Orringer MB, Sloan H. Esophagectomy without thoracotomy. J Thorac Cardiovasc Surg. 1978;76:643–54.
9. Mori K, Yamagata Y, Aikou S, et al. Short-term outcomes of robotic radical esophagectomy for esophageal cancer by a nontransthoracic approach compared with conventional transthoracic surgery. Dis Esophagus. 2016;29:429–34.
10. Hsu PK, Huang CS, Wu YC, Chou TY, Hsu WH. Open versus thoracoscopic esophagectomy in patients with esophageal squamous cell carcinoma. World J Surg. 2014;38:402–9.
11. Osugi H, Takemura M, Higashino M, Takada N, Lee S, Kinoshita H. A comparison of video-assisted thoracoscopic oesophagectomy and radical lymph node dissection for squamous cell cancer of the oesophagus with open operation. Br J Surg. 2003;90:108–13.
12. Daiko H, Nishimura M. A pilot study of the technical and oncologic feasibility of thoracoscopic esophagectomy with extended lymph node dissection in the prone position for clinical stage I thoracic esophageal carcinoma. Surg Endosc. 2012;26:673–80.
13. Tapias LF, Mathisen DJ, Wright CD, et al. Outcomes with open and minimally invasive Ivor Lewis esophagectomy after neoadjuvant therapy. Ann Thorac Surg. 2016;101:1097–103.
14. Miyasaka D, Okushiba S, Sasaki T, et al. Clinical evaluation of the feasibility of minimally invasive surgery in esophageal cancer. Asian J Endosc Surg. 2013;6:26–32.
15. Takeuchi H, Kawakubo H, Kitagawa Y. Current status of minimally invasive esophagectomy for patients with esophageal cancer. Gen Thorac Cardiovasc Surg. 2013;61:513–21.
16. Seesing MF, Gisbertz SS, Goense L, et al. A propensity score matched analysis of open versus minimally invasive transthoracic esophagectomy in the Netherlands. Ann Surg. 2017;266:839–46.
17. Mamidanna R, Bottle A, Aylin P, Faiz O, Hanna GB. Short-term outcomes following open versus minimally invasive esophagectomy for cancer in England: a population-based national study. Ann Surg. 2012;255:197–203.
18. Takeuchi H, Miyata H, Ozawa S, et al. Comparison of short-term outcomes between open and minimally invasive esophagectomy for esophageal cancer using a nationwide database in Japan. Ann Surg Oncol. 2017;24:1821–7.
19. Biere SS, van Berge Henegouwen MI, Maas KW, et al. Minimally invasive versus open oesophagectomy for patients with oesophageal cancer: a multicentre, open-label, randomised controlled trial. Lancet. 2012;379:1887–92.

Video-Assisted Thoracoscopic Surgery Intrathoracic Anastomosis Technique—The Extracorporeal Anastomosis Technique

11

Yong Won Seong

Abstract

The extracorporeal anastomosis technique for video-assisted thoracoscopic surgery (VATS) intrathoracic esophagogastric anastomosis is a convenient, easy technique to use in VATS esophagectomy. The surgeon can assess the viability and the status of the gastric conduit, and the introduction of a circular stapler can be easily done under direct vision extracorporeally, enabling easy and simple VATS intrathoracic anastomosis between the esophagus and the gastric conduit.

Keywords

Esophageal neoplasms · Minimally invasive surgery · Anastomosis · Video-assisted thoracic surgery

11.1 Introduction

Since Cuschieri et al. [1] reported the first series of five cases of minimally invasive esophagectomy (MIE), MIE has become an established and widely accepted approach for treating esophageal malignancies over the past two decades. It has been reported that when MIE is performed at high-volume centers, it shows similar clinical outcomes in terms of morbidity, mortality, and other oncologic outcomes to those of open esophagectomy, with clear advantages due to the minimally invasive approach [2]. Although MIE is technically demanding and involves a definite learning curve for surgeons, it is nonetheless an excellent approach for esophagectomy. The advantages of the minimally invasive approach include less postoperative pain and blood loss, a reduced incidence of pulmonary complications, and shorter hospital stays [3–5]. MIE techniques have been developed and evolved significantly from the initially used hybrid approaches (thoracoscopy combined with laparotomy or laparoscopy combined with thoracoscopy) to the totally minimally invasive approaches (thoracoscopy combined with laparoscopy, totally robotic) in current use. The esophagogastric anastomosis can be placed at cervical or intrathoracic location. The cervical anastomosis has been reported to pose a higher risk of anastomotic leakage, stricture, recurrent laryngeal nerve injury, and swallowing dysfunction, but with less severe morbidity from any leakage that does occur [6–8]. In contrast, transthoracic anastomosis has been reported to have more morbid consequences when an anastomotic leakage occurs [9]. When the 3-field MIE McKeown oper-

Y. W. Seong (✉)
Department of Thoracic and Cardiovascular Surgery, Seoul Metropolitan Government-Seoul National University Boramae Medical Center, Seoul National University College of Medicine, Seoul, Republic of Korea
e-mail: arqjoker@snu.ac.kr

K. Kim et al. (eds.), *Techniques in Minimally Invasive Thoracic Surgery*,
https://doi.org/10.1007/978-981-19-2472-9_11

ation is performed, every surgeon can assess the viability of the gastric conduit under direct vision. However, when the MIE Ivor Lewis operation is performed, direct visual assessment of the gastric conduit is very difficult, as it relies only on the quality of the thoracoscopic vision. Therefore, some reports have described successfully assessing gastric conduit viability by using fluorescence dyes such as indocyanine green [10–12]. However, these novel techniques of assessing gastric conduit viability by using novel imaging systems are not always available at relatively small-volume centers, and this discrepancy may explain why better clinical outcomes have been reported from large-volume centers. We would like to introduce a hybrid Ivor Lewis MIE technique (thoracoscopy combined with laparotomy) for video-assisted thoracoscopic surgery (VATS) extracorporeal intrathoracic esophagogastric anastomosis that can be easily performed and enables surgeons to assess the viability of the gastric conduit under direct vision.

11.2 Preoperative Workup and Planning

The preoperative workup is not different from that of patients undergoing open esophagectomy. Esophagogastroduodenoscopy is always performed to confirm the precise location of the tumor, its proximal and distal margins, the presence of Barrett esophagus, and the status of the stomach for the conduit. Computed tomography of the chest and abdomen, endoscopic ultrasonography, positron emission tomography–computed tomography, pulmonary function testing, and a cardiac function evaluation are performed. Patients with advanced clinical stages who have undergone neoadjuvant treatments (chemotherapy or chemoradiation) are also similarly prepared. Patients with upper esophageal cancers undergo the McKeown operation and are not candidates for this technique. Smoking cessation for 2 weeks or more is mandatory for every patient to minimize postoperative pulmonary complications. Antiplatelet agents such as aspirin or clopidogrel are stopped 5 days before surgery.

11.3 Operative Techniques

Anesthesia

All anesthetic procedures are performed or supervised by anesthesiologists who have experienced 100 or more esophagectomy cases. For all patients, endotracheal intubation for single-lung ventilation is performed with a left-sided double-lumen endotracheal tube (Shiley endotracheal tube; Medtronic, Minneapolis, MN, USA). The diameter of the double-lumen tube is determined according to the inner diameter of the left main bronchus of the patient on preoperative computed tomography. Patients are monitored with pulse oximetry, electrocardiography, and invasive and non-invasive measurements of arterial blood pressure. Central venous catheter insertion is not mandatory, and is mostly performed only in patients with advanced tumor stages or patients who have undergone neoadjuvant chemoradiation. A nasogastric Levin tube is always placed before surgery.

Abdominal Phase: Gastric Mobilization

The patient is placed in the supine position. The arms can be abducted or not. The surgeon operates on the right side of the patient.

The abdomen is mapped, and a midline laparotomy incision is made from below the xiphoid process to the umbilicus. The abdomen is thoroughly staged by inspecting and palpating the liver, peritoneum, and omentum to rule out any metastatic disease. A large wound protector with an OmniFlex retractor (Gadelius Medical K.K., Tokyo, Japan) affords an excellent surgical field (Fig. 11.1).

After identifying the gastrocolic omentum, the lesser sac is entered by creating a window at the greater omentum. Division of the omental branches of the gastroepiploic artery is performed. The right gastroepiploic arcade can be identified clearly by inspection and palpation, and must be protected securely during this procedure.

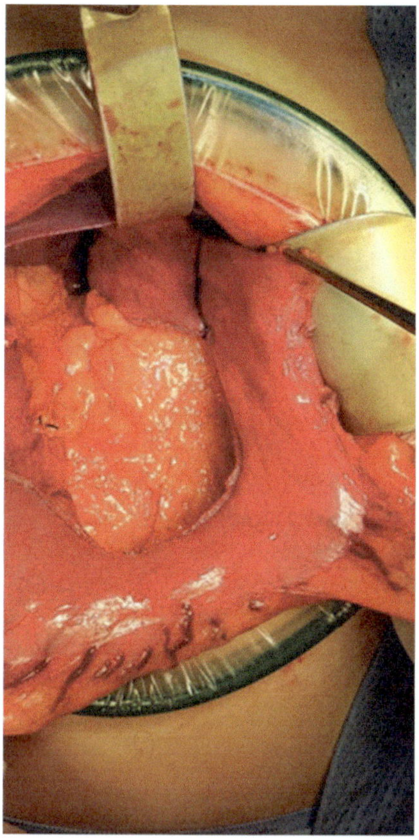

Fig. 11.1 Surgical view of midline laparotomy and gastric tube formation. Note that the 4-cm length of the uppermost fundus is left intact, not fully divided

Dissection is continued along the greater curve of the stomach until the gastroepiploic arcade ends, and then division of the short gastric vessels is performed using energy devices: ultrasonic shears (Harmonic HD 1000i; Ethicon, Raritan, NJ, USA) or bipolar devices (LigaSure; Medtronic). Especially when dividing the short gastric vessels by these energy devices, making the division closer right next to the gastric conduit is helpful for minimizing unsuspected bleeding after division with an energy device. Retrogastric attachments are divided after completing the division of the short gastric vessels.

Dissection of the pyloroantral region must be carefully and meticulously done because any injury to the proximal right gastroepiploic artery can result in a very frustrating situation. A partial or complete Kocher maneuver is sometimes needed for adequate mobilization.

The gastrohepatic ligament is opened. Triangular resection of the gastrohepatic ligament is helpful, affording adequate access for sweeping the lymph nodes (LNs) and fatty tissue, including the celiac LNs, left gastric LNs, and LNs along the splenic artery and the superior border of the pancreas. The left gastric artery and vein can be easily identified and dissected after this LN dissection. The left gastric artery and vein are divided after proximal double-ligation or double clipping using Weck Hem-o-Lok clips (Teleflex, Morrisville, NC, USA).

Dissection of the crus and mobilization of the distal abdominal esophagus are performed. The distal esophagus is retracted anteriorly, posteriorly, and bilaterally, and it then can be easily mobilized. Division of the crus is helpful for subsequent passage of the gastric conduit. A width of 3 fingerbreadths is adequate for most of the gastric conduit passage. At this point, the distal esophagus, gastric fundus, and antrum should be completely freely mobilized.

Abdominal Phase: Gastric Tube Formation

The Levin tube is requested to be withdrawn until 20 cm at the nasal orifice. The gastric tubing is performed before the pyloric drainage procedure (pyloromyotomy/pyloroplasty) and feeding jejunostomy, providing time to assess the viability of the gastric conduit.

The stomach is well stretched by the hands of the surgeon and the first assistant, and then the stomach is first divided across the antrum with an endoscopic purple stapler (Endo-GIA 60 mm Reload with Tri-staple Technology; Medtronic) or an endoscopic green stapler (Ethicon+Stapler with GST Reloads; Ethicon). When using the Ethicon stapler, we always hold the jaws in place for 15 s prior to firing for better compression and staple formation.

The subsequent stapling continues toward the fundus, maintaining a conduit width of 4–5 cm, parallel to the greater curvature. The stapling finishes with 4 cm of the fundus left intact, which later becomes an extracorporeal passage route for an EEA Circular Stapler (Medtronic). This site eventually needs to be stapled intrathoracically in the thoracic phase, so this area is marked with a surgical marker pen anteriorly and posteriorly (Fig. 11.1).

Reinforcing seromuscular sutures can be made along the stapler line, according to the surgeon's preference. We prefer to make seromuscular sutures at least at every junction of the stapler lines.

Abdominal Phase: Pyloric Drainage Procedures and Feeding Jejunostomy

Any pyloric drainage procedure—pyloromyotomy, pyloroplasty, or botulinum toxin injection—can be performed following the surgeon's preference. We usually perform a pyloromyotomy with an electrocautery amplitude of 5–10. The innermost layer of the pyloric muscle is divided by carefully removing the muscle fibers with a mosquito clamp, rather than by dividing the muscle through electrocautery.

Feeding jejunostomy tube insertion can be also performed according to the surgeon's preference. We usually perform feeding jejunostomy tube insertion in a Witzel fashion.

The laparotomy wound closure is performed layer-by-layer. We usually do not place any intraabdominal drains such as a Jackson–Pratt drain.

Thoracoscopic Phase (VATS Phase): Positioning and Port Placement

The patient is repositioned into the left lateral decubitus position for the thoracoscopic phase. The location of the double-lumen tube is reconfirmed by the anesthesiologist. The operating surgeon stands on the right side of the patient, while the assistant stands on the left side of the table.

Four thoracoscopic ports are used. The right scapula and the locations for the ports are shown in Fig. 11.2a. A 5-cm utility incision is made on the fifth rib on the anterior axillary line, and then a 4-cm segment of the fifth rib is resected using a periosteal elevator and a rib cutter (Fig. 11.2b). Sharp resection margins of the ribs are made blunt by using a rongeur. A 14-mm incision is made on the seventh intercostal space, along the midaxillary line, for a 12-mm trocar. A 7-mm incision is made on the sixth intercostal space, anterior to the scapular tip, for a 5-mm trocar. Finally, a 12-mm incision is made on the third intercostal space, along the anterior axillary line, for a 10-mm trocar, which is used as an assistant port. The completed port placement is shown in Fig. 11.2c.

Thoracoscopic Phase (VATS Phase): Esophagectomy and LN Dissection

The mediastinal pleura is vertically opened along the course of the esophagus. The azygous vein is divided using a vascular endoscopic stapler. The posterior stump of the divided azygous vein is sutured to the posterior mediastinal pleura with a 3-0 silk suture, and the suture is then tacked and clipped with a 5-mm Weck Hem-o-Lok. This affords a better surgical view of the esophagus. This tacking suture is later removed before wound closure.

Esophagectomy using an energy device is performed. Whether or not to remove the entire mesoesophagus, including the thoracic duct, relies on the surgeon's preference. We usually keep the thoracic duct intact. After finishing esophagectomy, complete total 2-field LN dissection is performed. The bilateral paraesophageal, bilateral recurrent laryngeal, subcarinal, hilar, and aortopulmonary window LNs are completely removed.

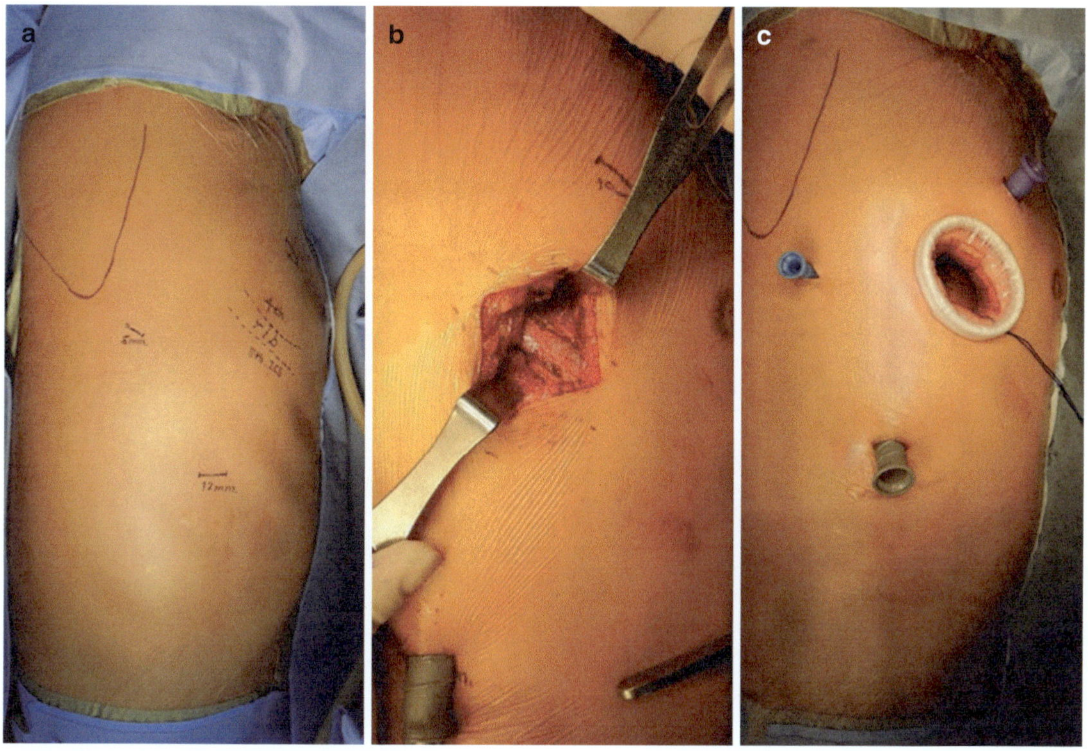

Fig. 11.2 (**a**) The location of the ports to be placed is shown by a marker pen. (**b**) A 4-cm segment of the fifth rib is resected for subsequent easy passage of the extracorporeal procedures. (**c**) Image after the port placement

Thoracoscopic Phase (VATS Phase): Extracorporeal Introduction of the Circular Stapler

A purse-string suture is made at the upper thoracic esophagus over the azygous vein level with a 2-0 polyester suture (Ethibond EXCEL; Ethicon). Then, a vertical esophagotomy incision is made 5–10 mm below the purse-string suture. The anvil for a 28-mm or 25-mm circular stapler (EEA Circular Stapler; Medtronic) is vertically inserted into the esophagotomy. The anvil is then introduced into the upper thoracic esophagus through the purse-string suture. When introducing the anvil upward, keeping the anvil vertically while pushing the anvil upward enables us to pass the anvil through the purse-string suture more easily (Fig. 11.3). After the anvil passes the purse-string suture, the anvil is rotated, and then the suture is tied down.

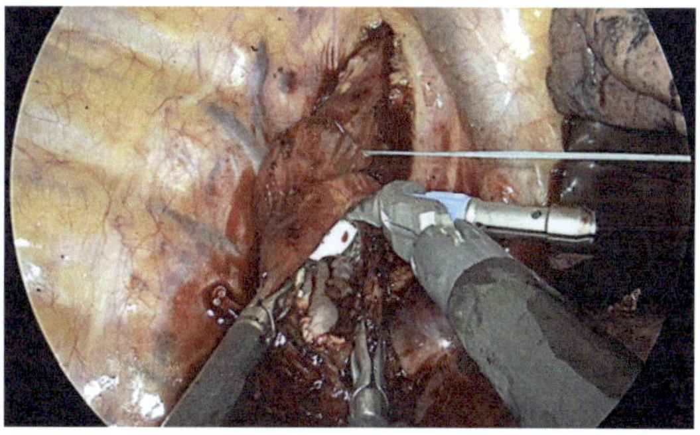

Fig. 11.3 Intrathoracic anvil insertion is shown. Gentle vertical upward introduction of the anvil, not rotating below the purse-string suture, is important for easier passage of the anvil through the purse-string suture

The proximal esophagus is divided right below the previously tied-down purse-string suture, then is brought out extracorporeally through the utility incision and tied down with a 2-0 silk ligature.

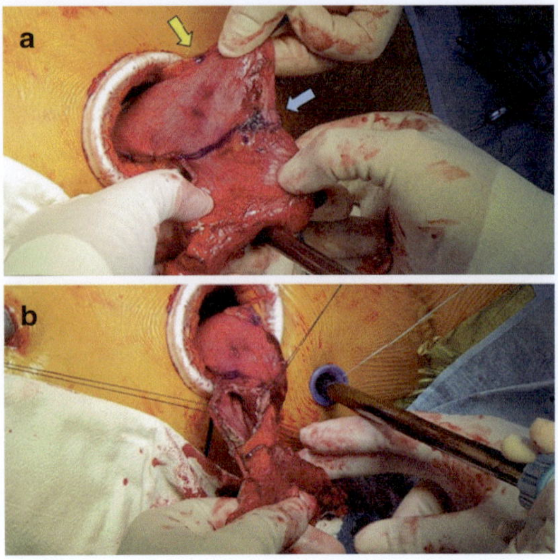

Fig. 11.4 The gastric conduit is extracted through the utility incision, followed by (**a**) extracorporeal assessment of the conduit and (**b**) gastrotomy with tacking sutures for introducing the EEA stapler (Medtronic, Minneapolis, MN, USA). Note the 4-cm distance between the yellow and blue arrows in (**a**). Keeping this distance between the circular stapler line and the linear stapler line is important for preventing anastomosis site ischemia and leakage

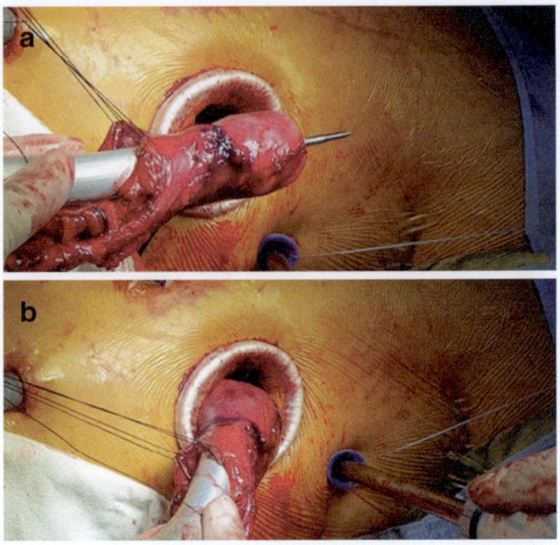

Fig. 11.5 An EEA stapler (Medtronic, Minneapolis, MN, USA) is inserted extracorporeally through the gastrotomy (**a**), and then reintroduced through the utility incision (**b**). With the previous segmental fifth-rib resection, this procedure can be easily performed without any difficulty in passage

The gastric conduit is pulled up into the thoracic cavity under thoracoscopic vision, and is then brought out extracorporeally through the utility incision. At this stage, the surgeon can assess the viability of the gastric conduit under direct vision. The surgeon can identify the line that was previously marked during the abdominal phase. This line later will become the final stapler line after finishing the EEA stapling. The EEA stapler puncture site is shown by a yellow arrow in Fig. 11.4a. We keep at least a 4-cm distance between this puncture site and the final stapling line in order to maximize the submucosal blood flow around the circular stapling site to prevent anastomotic leakage (Fig. 11.4a). A 4-cm gastrotomy incision is made right next to the stapler line at the remnant fundus. The gastric and esophageal blood and contents are removed by a sucker, and each opened side of the fundus is then tacked with a 2-0 silk suture (Fig. 11.4b).

An EEA stapler is introduced through the gastrotomy, and the fundus is then punctured (Fig. 11.5a). The punctured gastric conduit and the EEA can be easily and smoothly reintroduced into the thoracic cavity through the utility incision. The previous segmental resection of the fifth rib affords adequate space for these extracorporeal procedures. It is important to gently pull the previously placed 2 silk tacking sutures to maintain the EEA at the proper position inside the conduit (Fig. 11.5b).

Thoracoscopic Phase (VATS Phase): Intrathoracic Anastomosis

With the reintroduction of the conduit intrathoracically, the VATS camera affords an excellent view of the previously placed anvil and the introduction of the EEA and the conduit (Fig. 11.6a). Once the sharp end of the EEA tip enters the anvil, the cervical vertebra and the thoracic inlet serve as a supporting wall; therefore, docking between the main EEA body and the anvil can be easily performed (Fig. 11.6b). After stapling is finished, the EEA and the anvil are gently retrieved and the donut-shaped margins of the cross section at the removed anvil are inspected for completeness and sent to the pathologist for a frozen section.

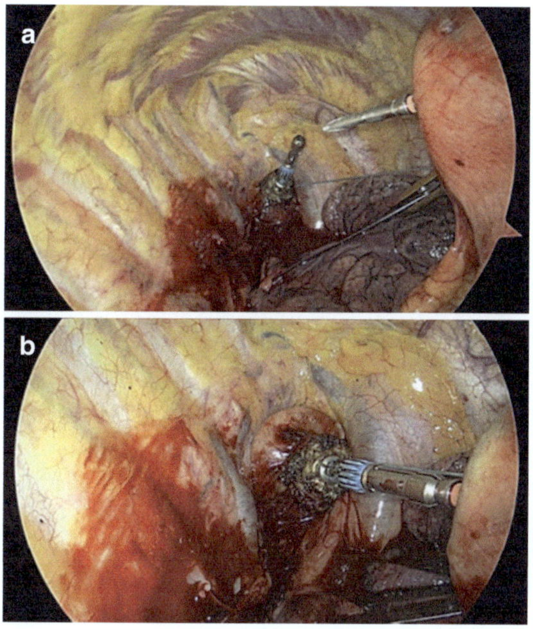

Fig. 11.6 Video-assisted thoracoscopic surgery intrathoracic anastomosis is performed (**a**). With the cervical vertebra and the small thoracic inlet serving as a supporting table, docking between the anvil and the body of the EEA stapler (Medtronic, Minneapolis, MN, USA) can be easily done (**b**)

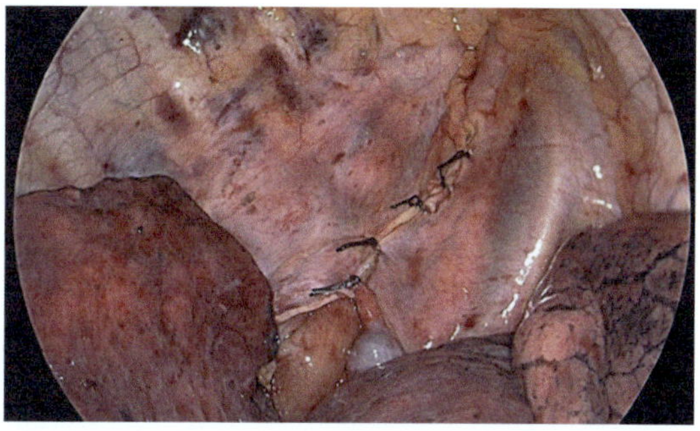

Fig. 11.7 The upper portion of the mediastinal pleura over the azygous vein level is suture-repaired with multiple interrupted 3-0 silk sutures. This closure of the upper pleura is an easy procedure that takes only a couple of minutes, and serves as a viable tissue barrier around the anastomosis site

The surgeon can check the completeness of the anastomosis by entering the thoracoscope through the gastrotomy site where the EEA entered, but this is not routinely performed. The previously marked linear line on the conduit is stapled with the same endoscopic stapler loads that were used for conduit formation.

The nasogastric Levin tube is now reinserted and fixed at 45 cm at the nasal orifice. This usually results in an adequate location of the tip of the nasogastric tube, just above the pylorus. Multiple interrupted seromuscular sutures (3-0 silk sutures) are made over the final linear stapled line.

Repair of the upper mediastinal pleura is always performed using multiple interrupted 3-0 silk sutures (Fig. 11.7). We consider this procedure very important, since this closure of the pleura—especially around the anastomosis site—provides protection from viable tissue, and even if there is a leakage postoperatively it can be successfully treated by endoluminal vacuum-assisted closure therapy, with the closed mediastinal pleura serving as a viable flap layer. The previously tacked posterior azygous vein stump is released.

The gastric conduit below the azygous vein is adequately adjusted; if there is any redundancy, the redundant portion is put back into the abdominal cavity. When an adequate position of the conduit is confirmed, the conduit is fixed to the posterior mediastinal pleura with 3 or 4 interrupted 3-0 silk sutures.

Irrigation of the thoracic cavity with warm distilled water is done. A single 28 F straight soft straight chest tube is inserted, and wound closure is performed layer-by-layer. The patient is extubated and transferred to the intensive care unit.

11.4 Discussion

Lateral Decubitus Versus Prone Position

Luketich et al. [13] reported a large series of total MIE (thoracoscopy combined with laparoscopy) in 222 patients with impressive clinical outcomes, including low mortality and pulmonary complication rates of 1.4% and 7.7%, respectively. In this series, all the cases were performed with the patients in the lateral decubitus position, as was done for most MIE procedures in this period [13].

However, there were concerns regarding pulmonary complications, as the lateral decubitus requires complete lung collapse and therefore often causes serious pulmonary complications. Palanivelu et al. [14] reported a large series of thoracoscopic mobilization of the esophagus in the prone position with excellent clinical outcomes, as shown by mortality and pulmonary complication rates of 1.54% and 1.54%, respectively. In their systematic review and pooled analysis, Markar et al. [15] reported that prone MIE is superior to the lateral decubitus position, with reduced pulmonary complications, lower estimated blood loss, and increased LN harvest. However, urgent conversion to lateral thoracotomy is difficult when the patient is in the prone position. Therefore, a modified semiprone position was reported and adopted by many surgeons [16]. In our technique, we perform the procedure with the patient in the lateral decubitus position, but we never grab or clamp the lung for traction. We only add gentle pushing to the lung with an endoscopic fan retractor or an endoscopic peanut.

Hand-Sewn Versus Side-to-Side Linear Stapling Versus End-to-End Circular Stapling

In the days of open esophagectomy, the hand-sewn anastomosis was preferred by many surgeons, with good results [17]. There have been many reports describing favorable clinical outcomes of hand-sewn MIE performed using a robot, with the aid of the articulating robotic arms and the three-dimensional imaging system [18]. However, there have not been many reports of minimally invasive hand-sewn anastomosis due to its technical difficulty with instruments without articulation [19, 20].

The linear stapling technique is a side-to-side anastomosis between the esophagus and the conduit, which has been reported to be functionally favorable with a larger diameter of the anastomosis that offers easy passage of the intraluminal content and reduced circular pressure at the anastomosis site. These factors might explain the low incidence of anastomotic leakage and strictures [21–23].

Since Fain et al. [24] reported the first use of a circular stapling apparatus in colorectal cancer surgery in 1975, the device and the technique have evolved. Since this technique is the longest-known and best-developed, it is well-standardized and relatively easy to learn. However, there are still many technically important points, and the learning curve is steep for novice surgeons. For example, inserting an EEA anvil thoracoscopically is very difficult if the proximal esophagus is completely divided. Vertical esophagotomy below the purse-string suture and an upward vertical entrance of the EEA anvil is a technique that almost always makes the insertion of a 28-mm anvil possible. It is also very important to minimize the size of the tied esophageal stump of the anvil before docking of the EEA. If the tied esophageal stump is large, it can be squeezed out laterally between the stapler lines when docking, which can result in an area of incomplete stapling.

Extracorporeal Anastomosis Versus Intracorporeal Anastomosis

Extracorporeal anastomosis is a well-known and established concept in the area of general surgery. For example, right-side hemicolectomy for right colonic cancer is commonly performed [25], and laparoscopic-assisted right hemicolectomy with an extracorporeal anastomosis is the standard technique in most countries. The current standard procedure for laparoscopic extracorporeal anastomosis requires adequate positioning of the utility incision, mobilization of the colon, and mesenteric traction in order to extract the ileum and ascending colon; this can result in surgical trauma, leading to postoperative morbidities such as prolonged ileus, pain associated with pulmonary function, and wound infection with a prolonged length of stay [25–27]. Furthermore, the extracorporeal anastomosis technique for laparoscopic-assisted right hemicolectomy requires the location of the extraction wound to be in the upper/mid-abdomen, which is known to result in increased postoperative pain when compared with the wound located in the lower abdomen [27]. Van Oostendorp et al. [28] reported in their meta-analysis that intracorporeal anastomosis was associated with less morbidity and a shorter length of stay, suggesting that it enabled a faster recovery than occurred after extracorporeal anastomosis.

Although extracorporeal anastomosis is reported to have limitations compared with intracorporeal anastomosis in right hemicolectomy, the extracorporeal anastomosis technique in VATS intrathoracic anastomosis after esophagectomy is different. The location of the utility incision is not different from that of the conventional VATS intracorporeal anastomosis technique. No additional mobilization of the gastric conduit or Kocher maneuver is required to extract the conduit. The surgeon can thoroughly assess the viability of the conduit under direct vision and palpation, and the introduction of the EEA and final conduit design can also be accurately planned extracorporeally. Kim et al. [29] reported 66 patients with esophageal cancer who underwent VATS Ivor Lewis operations using the extracorporeal anastomosis technique. They presented excellent clinical outcomes without any anastomotic leakage or stricture.

11.5 Conclusion

Extracorporeal anastomosis for VATS intrathoracic esophagogastric anastomosis is a convenient, easy technique without any requirement for a robotic system, articulating instruments, or any other novel devices or instruments; therefore, this technique can be learned and adopted by surgeons who are newly starting to perform MIE.

Conflict of Interest No potential conflict of interest relevant to this article was reported.

References

1. Cuschieri A, Shimi S, Banting S. Endoscopic oesophagectomy through a right thoracoscopic approach. J R Coll Surg Edinb. 1992;37:7–11.
2. Levy RM, Trivedi D, Luketich JD. Minimally invasive esophagectomy. Surg Clin N Am. 2012;92:1265–85.
3. Xiong WL, Li R, Lei HK, Jiang ZY. Comparison of outcomes between minimally invasive oesophagectomy and open oesophagectomy for oesophageal cancer. ANZ J Surg. 2017;87:165–70.
4. Nagpal K, Ahmed K, Vats A, et al. Is minimally invasive surgery beneficial in the management of esophageal cancer? A meta-analysis. Surg Endosc. 2010;24:1621–9.
5. Verhage RJ, Hazebroek EJ, Boone J, van Hillegersberg R. Minimally invasive surgery compared to open procedures in esophagectomy for cancer: a systematic review of the literature. Minerva Chir. 2009;64:135–46.
6. Martin RE, Letsos P, Taves DH, Inculet RI, Johnston H, Preiksaitis HG. Oropharyngeal dysphagia in esophageal cancer before and after transhiatal esophagectomy. Dysphagia. 2001;16:23–31.
7. Hulscher JB, Tijssen JG, Obertop H, van Lanschot JJ. Transthoracic versus transhiatal resection for carcinoma of the esophagus: a meta-analysis. Ann Thorac Surg. 2001;72:306–13.
8. Easterling CS, Bousamra M 2nd, Lang IM, et al. Pharyngeal dysphagia in postesophagectomy patients: correlation with deglutitive biomechanics. Ann Thorac Surg. 2000;69:989–92.
9. Hulscher JB, van Sandick JW, de Boer AG, et al. Extended transthoracic resection compared with limited transhiatal resection for adenocarcinoma of the esophagus. N Engl J Med. 2002;347:1662–9.
10. Luo RJ, Zhu ZY, He ZF, Xu Y, Wang YZ, Chen P. Efficacy of indocyanine green fluorescence angiography in preventing anastomotic leakage after McKeown minimally invasive esophagectomy. Front Oncol. 2021;10:619822.
11. Ladak F, Dang JT, Switzer N, et al. Indocyanine green for the prevention of anastomotic leaks following esophagectomy: a meta-analysis. Surg Endosc. 2019;33:384–94.
12. Schlottmann F, Patti MG. Evaluation of gastric conduit perfusion during esophagectomy with indocyanine green fluorescence imaging. J Laparoendosc Adv Surg Tech A. 2017;27:1305–8.
13. Luketich JD, Alvelo-Rivera M, Buenaventura PO, et al. Minimally invasive esophagectomy: outcomes in 222 patients. Ann Surg. 2003;238:486–95.
14. Palanivelu C, Prakash A, Senthilkumar R, et al. Minimally invasive esophagectomy: thoracoscopic mobilization of the esophagus and mediastinal lymphadenectomy in prone position: experience of 130 patients. J Am Coll Surg. 2006;203:7–16.
15. Markar SR, Wiggins T, Antonowicz S, Zacharakis E, Hanna GB. Minimally invasive esophagectomy: lateral decubitus vs. prone positioning; systematic review and pooled analysis. Surg Oncol. 2015;24:212–9.
16. Seesing MF, Goense L, Ruurda JP, Luyer MD, Nieuwenhuijzen GA, van Hillegersberg R. Minimally invasive esophagectomy: a propensity score-matched analysis of semiprone versus prone position. Surg Endosc. 2018;32:2758–65.
17. Cerfolio RJ, Bryant AS, Canon CL, Dhawan R, Eloubeidi MA. Is botulinum toxin injection of the pylorus during Ivor Lewis [corrected] esophagogas-

trectomy the optimal drainage strategy? J Thorac Cardiovasc Surg. 2009;137:565–72.
18. Plat VD, Stam WT, Schoonmade LJ, Heineman DJ, van der Peet DL, Daams F. Implementation of robot-assisted Ivor Lewis procedure: robotic hand-sewn, linear or circular technique? Am J Surg. 2020;220:62–8.
19. Cadiere GB, Dapri G, Himpens J, Fodderie L, Rajan A. Ivor Lewis esophagectomy with manual esogastric anastomosis by thoracoscopy in prone position and laparoscopy. Surg Endosc. 2010;24:1482–5.
20. Watson DI, Davies N, Jamieson GG. Totally endoscopic Ivor Lewis esophagectomy. Surg Endosc. 1999;13:293–7.
21. Yanni F, Singh P, Tewari N, et al. Comparison of outcomes with semi-mechanical and circular stapled intrathoracic esophagogastric anastomosis following esophagectomy. World J Surg. 2019;43:2483–9.
22. Ben-David K, Tuttle R, Kukar M, Rossidis G, Hochwald SN. Minimally invasive esophagectomy utilizing a stapled side-to-side anastomosis is safe in the western patient population. Ann Surg Oncol. 2016;23:3056–62.
23. Deng XF, Liu QX, Zhou D, Min JX, Dai JG. Hand-sewn vs linearly stapled esophagogastric anastomosis for esophageal cancer: a meta-analysis. World J Gastroenterol. 2015;21:4757–64.
24. Fain SN, Patin CS, Morgenstern L. Use of a mechanical suturing apparatus in low colorectal anastomosis. Arch Surg. 1975;110:1079–82.
25. Van Leersum NJ, Snijders HS, Henneman D, et al. The Dutch surgical colorectal audit. Eur J Surg Oncol. 2013;39:1063–70.
26. Kennedy RH, Francis EA, Wharton R, et al. Multicenter randomized controlled trial of conventional versus laparoscopic surgery for colorectal cancer within an enhanced recovery programme: EnROL. J Clin Oncol. 2014;32:1804–11.
27. Vlug MS, Wind J, Hollmann MW, et al. Laparoscopy in combination with fast track multimodal management is the best perioperative strategy in patients undergoing colonic surgery: a randomized clinical trial (LAFA-study). Ann Surg. 2011;254:868–75.
28. Van Oostendorp S, Elfrink A, Borstlap W, et al. Intracorporeal versus extracorporeal anastomosis in right hemicolectomy: a systematic review and meta-analysis. Surg Endosc. 2017;31:64–77.
29. Kim K, Park JS, Seo H. Early outcomes of video-assisted thoracic surgery (VATS) Ivor Lewis operation for esophageal squamous cell carcinoma: the extracorporeal anastomosis technique. Surg Laparosc Endosc Percutan Tech. 2013;23:303–8.

12 Robot-Assisted Thoracoscopic Esophagectomy with Total Mediastinal Lymphadenectomy: A Guide to a Systematic Approach Using the Concept of Fascial Plane Dissection

Byung Jo Park and Dae Joon Kim

Abstract

Recent case series and meta-analyses have suggested that robot-assisted minimally invasive esophagectomy (RAMIE) could be a useful alternative to video-assisted thoracic surgery esophagectomy. The advantages of RAMIE are a three-dimensional view, 7 degrees of freedom, and tremor filtering, which enable more meticulous lymph node dissection with a lower incidence of complications. However, in radical esophagectomy, understanding the concepts of the fascia and compartment is crucial for successful and reliable dissection. The first RAMIE in Korea was performed by our team in July 2006, and since then, we have developed related techniques to achieve better short- and long-term outcomes. The key step in RAMIE for esophageal squamous cell carcinoma is dissection of the upper mediastinum due to the difficulty of lymph node dissection and the high incidence of nodal metastasis in the area. Herein, we describe the technique of fascial plane dissection with esophageal suspension during RAMIE.

B. J. Park · D. J. Kim (✉)
Department of Thoracic and Cardiovascular Surgery, Severance Hospital, Yonsei University College of Medicine, Seoul, Republic of Korea
e-mail: kdjcool@yuhs.ac

Keywords

Esophagectomy · Robot-assisted · Lymph node dissection

12.1 Introduction

Since robot-assisted minimally invasive esophagectomy (RAMIE) was introduced in the mid-2000s, numerous case series and meta-analyses have suggested that it could be a useful alternative to video-assisted thoracic surgery esophagectomy (VATS-E). The currently used da Vinci Surgical System provides key functions such as three-dimensional vision, tremor filtering, motion scaling, and the endo-wrist function, which are expected to decrease the incidence of morbidity after RAMIE compared to that after VATS-E [1–4]. Since the first RAMIE in Korea, performed by our team (Severance Hospital) in July 2006, we have developed useful techniques for radical esophagectomy with favorable postoperative and oncologic outcomes [5–9]. Although novel devices and technologies have been introduced in the past decade, understanding the microanatomy of the esophagus and related structures is a prerequisite for the success of RAMIE. Here, we present in detail a systematic approach to RAMIE using fascial plane dissection.

K. Kim et al. (eds.), *Techniques in Minimally Invasive Thoracic Surgery*,
https://doi.org/10.1007/978-981-19-2472-9_12

12.2 Port Placement and Patient Position

After general endotracheal anesthesia with a bronchial blocker, the patient is turned to the semi-prone position (Fig. 12.1). An 8-mm port (P2) is placed at the sixth intercostal space (ICS), just below the inferior scapula tip, and a 30° thoracoscope is inserted. After an assessment for pleural seeding or adhesion, CO_2 gas is insufflated at a pressure of 8–10 mmHg. An 8-mm port (P1) is placed at the third or fourth ICS on the posterior axillary line (PAL). In the case illustrated here, the target area was the thoracic inlet; thus, a mark was drawn on a straight line from the camera port towards it. Then, an 8-mm port (P3) was inserted at the eighth or ninth ICS on the PAL, and another 8-mm port (P4) was inserted at the 11th ICS on the scapular tip line. A 12-mm accessory port (PA) was inserted at the fifth or sixth ICS on the anterior axillary line. The robotic cart (da Vinci Xi) was positioned at the patient's left side. A green target from a laser-guided system was aligned with P2, and the camera was inserted through P2, targeted at the thoracic inlet. The cart then automatically adjusted its boom in the optimized configuration, the remaining robotic arms were docked, and the rest of the instruments were inserted.

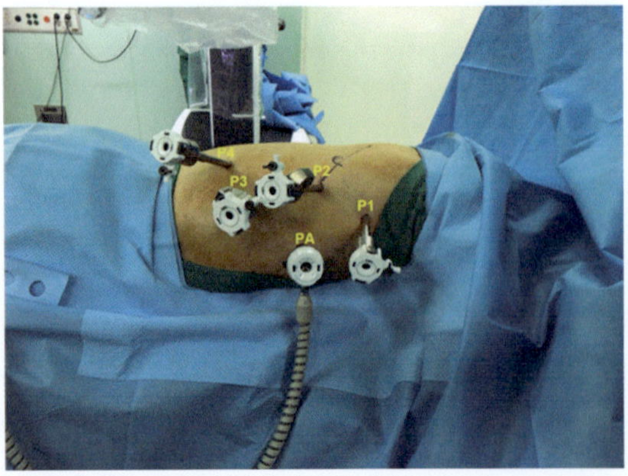

Fig. 12.1 Port placement and patient position for robot-assisted thoracoscopic esophagectomy: P1–P4 (8-mm port) and PA (12-mm accessory port)

12.3 Dissection of the Upper Mediastinum

Practical Anatomy of the Upper Mediastinum

Figure 12.2 shows a schematic diagram of the upper mediastinum, superior to the aortic arch. The visceral compartment contains the esophagus and trachea, while the vascular compartment contains the major arteries and veins. Each compartment is surrounded by thin connective tissue layers (the visceral and vascular fascia). The vagus nerve descends along the carotid artery in the vascular compartment. The recurrent laryngeal nerve (RLN) branches from the vagus nerve penetrate the visceral fascia and run upward along the trachea in the visceral compartment. The cardiac branch of the sympathetic nerve is in the vascular compartment, and the thoracic duct travels between the visceral and vascular fascia. To clear all the lymph nodes around the RLN without nerve injury, attention should be focused on the relationship between the visceral fascia and the RLN at the left side, as most cases of RLN palsy occur in this area.

There are two major routes of lymphatic metastasis in esophageal cancer [10–13]. Intramural metastasis mainly occurs through the longitudinal lymphatic channels in the submucosal layer, whereas extramural metastasis occurs through peri-esophageal lymphatics. Thus, it is essential to dissect all lymphatic tissues in the visceral compartment to achieve excellent locoregional control. Another route of metastasis is the thoracic duct and its surrounding nodes. The thoracic duct receives lymphatic flow from abdominal lymph nodes and direct drainage from the esophagus with a nodal relay. This suggests the possibility of rapid lymph drainage into the systemic circulation via the thoracic duct in esophageal cancer. Although the effect of thoracic duct resection has yet to be established, we routinely dissect the thoracic duct en bloc with the esophagus.

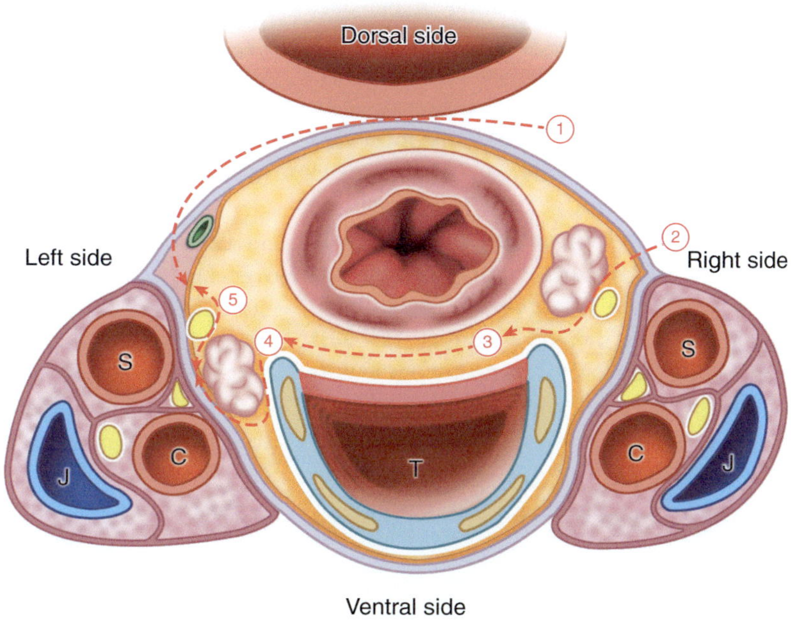

Fig. 12.2 Schematic drawing of the upper mediastinum superior to the aortic arch. Yellow line, visceral fascia; pink line, vascular fascia; yellow oval cross-section structures, nerve; green oval cross-section structure, thoracic duct; *E* esophagus, *T* trachea, *J* jugular vein, *S* subclavian artery, *C* common carotid artery; numbers and the red dotted line, dissection order

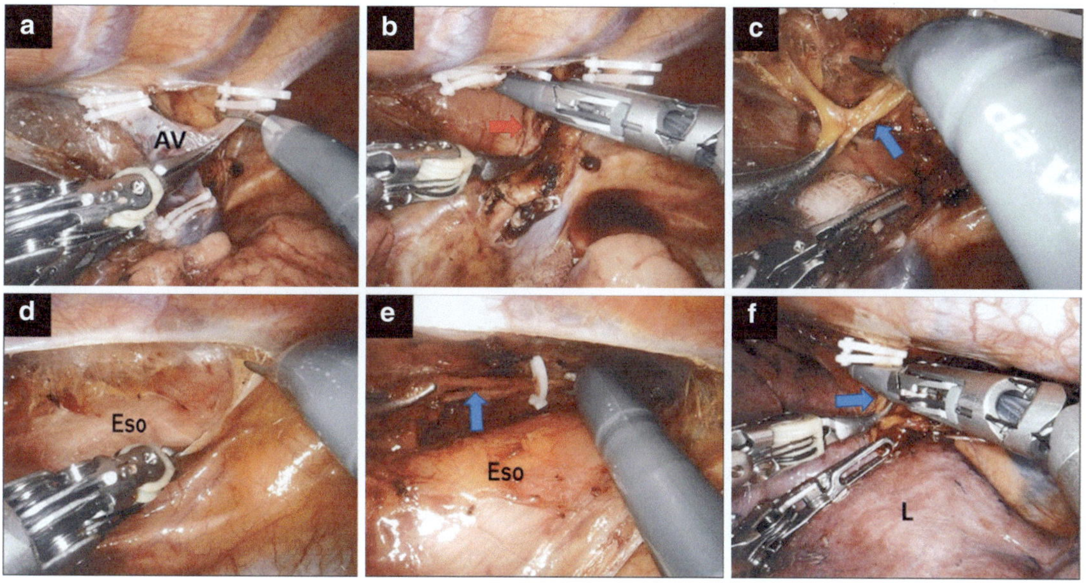

Fig. 12.3 Dissection of the dorsal part of the upper mediastinum. The thoracic duct is identified and resected after clipping. (**a**) Azygos vein (AV) division after applying Hem-o-lok clips. (**b**) Right bronchial artery division with vessel sealer extension. (**c**) Identification of the thoracic duct. (**d**) Dissection of the dorsal mediastinal pleura. (**e**, **f**) Resection of the thoracic duct. *Eso* esophagus, *L* lung; red arrow, right bronchial artery; blue arrow, thoracic duct

Dorsal Part Dissection

A ProGrasp forceps is inserted through P3 to compress the lung while pulling the esophagus down. Dissection is begun with a curved bipolar dissector (through P4) and monopolar curved scissors (through P1). The azygos vein is cut after applying Hem-o-lok clips (Fig. 12.3a); then, the right bronchial artery is identified and cut with a vessel sealer (Fig. 12.3b). For routine resection of the thoracic duct, identification of the duct below the azygos vein is the next step (Fig. 12.3c). The dorsal side of the mediastinal pleura is opened (Fig. 12.3d). The thoracic duct is resected from its cranial part (Fig. 12.3e) to the most caudal part, and the caudal end is cut after clipping to prevent chylothorax (Fig. 12.3f). The dorsal side of the esophagus is subsequently dissected with monopolar curved scissors, and the dorsolateral part of the esophagus is mobilized. The left subclavian artery need not be identified, as it is located outside the visceral compartment and its dissection with the energy device may cause thermal injury to the left RLN.

Ventral Part Dissection

A ProGrasp forceps is inserted through P4 to lift the esophagus, and a curved bipolar dissector is moved to P3. After lifting the esophagus, the right vagus nerve is identified, and the mediastinal pleura is opened towards the level of the subclavian artery (Fig. 12.4a). The vascular sheath over the right vagus nerve is opened, which allows identification of the right RLN, as it penetrates the visceral compartment in most patients (Fig. 12.4b). The visceral sheath over the right RLN is cut using curved scissors, along with the identified esophageal branches of the RLN

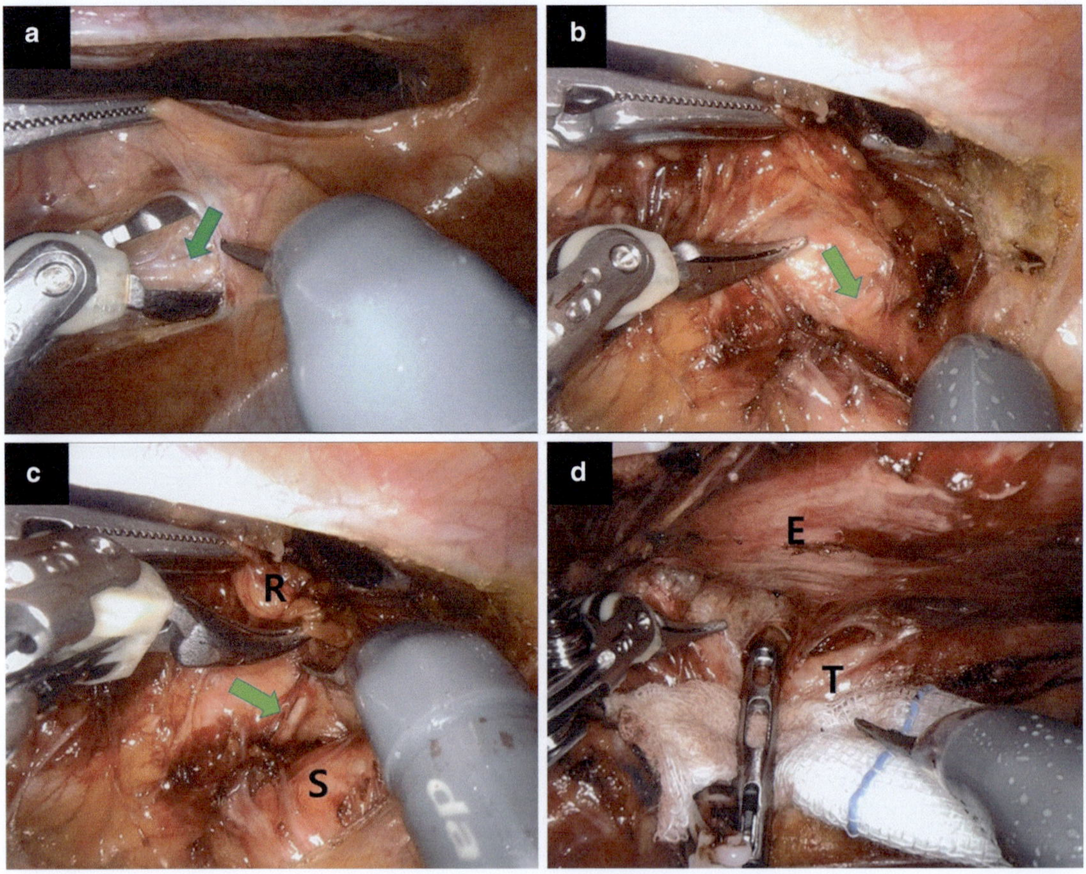

Fig. 12.4 Dissection of the ventral part of the upper mediastinum. Lymph nodes along the right recurrent laryngeal nerve (RLN) are dissected. (**a**) The mediastinal pleura above the vagus nerve is opened. (**b**) Identification of the right RLN penetrating into the visceral compartment. (**c**) Identification and incision of the esophageal branches of the RLN. (**d**) Mobilization of the esophagus from the trachea. *R* right RLN lymph nodes, *S* subclavian artery, *E* esophagus, *T* trachea; green arrow, vagus nerve; fluorescent green arrow, right RLN

(Fig. 12.4c). The lymphoadipose tissue posterior to the RLN is then dissected carefully.

The next step is to mobilize the esophagus from the trachea. The esophagus is lifted using a ProGrasp forceps (through P4), and the trachea is retracted to the right side with a grasper or a peanut dissector by an assistant (through PA) (Fig. 12.4d). The loose connective tissue between the esophageal muscle and the trachealis muscle is dissected, with careful avoidance of airway injury in the process. After the esophagus is completely mobilized from the trachea, the lymphoadipose tissue along the left lateral border of the trachea is dissected, and small vessels from the tracheoesophageal artery are cauterized with monopolar curved scissors. The visceral fascia, a shiny, glossy membrane-like structure that is the boundary of lymph node dissection in the upper mediastinum, can be identified underneath the lymphoadipose tissue.

Dissection Along the Left Recurrent Laryngeal Nerve

After identification of the visceral fascia, a single strand of nylon tape is applied to encircle the esophagus and tie it at three points (Figs. 12.5a and 12.6a). This maneuver, termed esophageal suspension, provides a wider operating space in the left paratracheal space while preventing nerve injury from excessive stretching or kinking during the procedure. Identification of the left RLN at the level of the tracheobronchial angle is the next step. After identification of the visceral fascia layer, the nerve can easily be identified as it is located just over the fascia, which appears like a curtain on a wall (Figs. 12.5b and 12.6b). Once the nerve is identified, the lymphoadipose tissue in the medial part is sharply dissected out from the nerve. At this point, the esophageal branches of the left RLN should not be cut to maintain

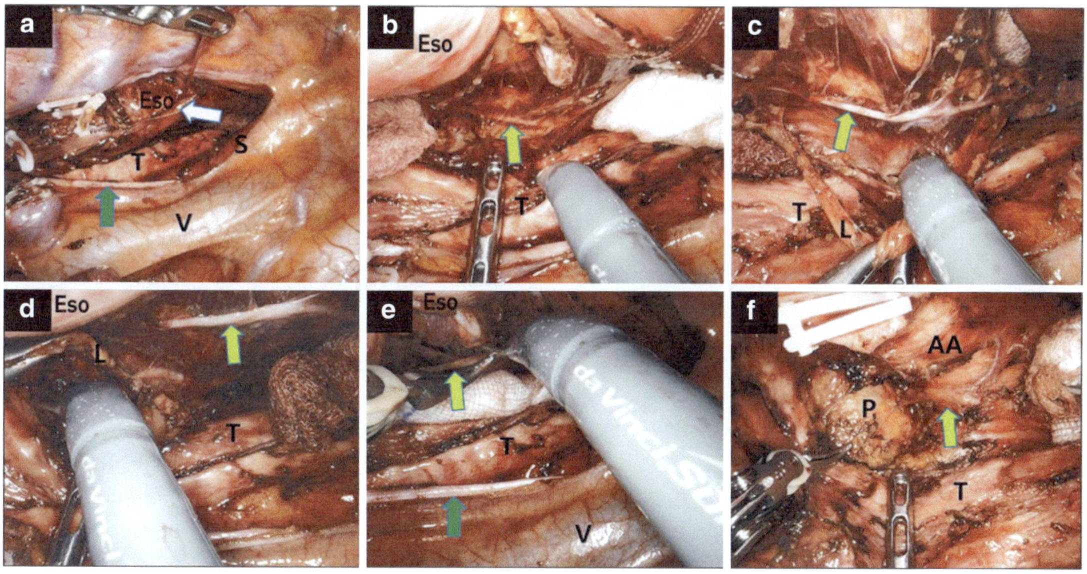

Fig. 12.5 Dissection along the left recurrent laryngeal nerve (RLN). (**a**) The esophagus is tied at 3 points using a single strand of nylon tape. (**b**) The left RLN is identified. (**c, d**) Left RLN lymph nodes are dissected. (**e**) The esophageal branches of the left RLN are cut. (**f**) Lymph nodes at the tracheobronchial angle and the infra-aortic area are dissected. *Eso* esophagus, *T* trachea, *S* subclavian artery, *V* superior vena cava, *L* left RLN lymph nodes, *AA* aortic arch, *P* left pulmonary artery; white arrow, nylon tape; green arrow, vagus nerve; fluorescent green arrow, left RLN

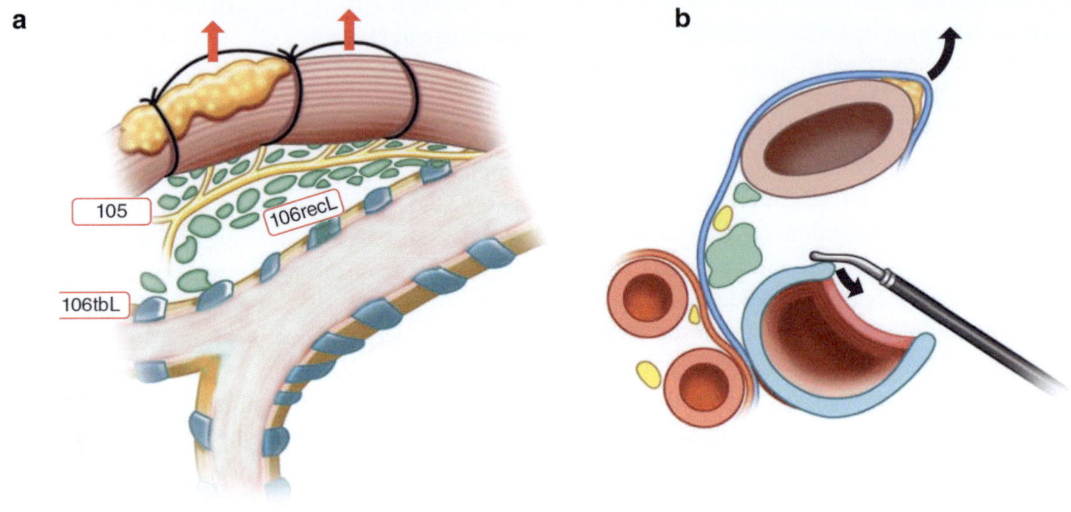

Fig. 12.6 Schematic drawing of dissection along the left recurrent laryngeal nerve (RLN). (**a**) Lateral view of the left RLN and lymph node station after the esophagus is retracted to the right side. (**b**) Transection view of the left RLN and lymph node station after the esophagus is retracted to the right side

esophageal suspension (Fig. 12.5c). All lymphatic tissues within the visceral fascia are carefully removed (Fig. 12.5d). Then, the esophageal branches of the left RLN are cut with scissors (Fig. 12.5e), and the visceral fascia between the nerve and the esophagus is cut to fully mobilize the esophagus. Lymph nodes at the tracheobronchial angle and the infra-aortic area are dissected completely until the left pulmonary artery is identifiable (Fig. 12.5f).

12.4 Middle to Lower Mediastinum Dissection

The dorsal side of the mediastinal pleura is opened along the ventral margin of the azygous vein. The next step is to dissect the duct (Fig. 12.7a) and lymphoadipose tissue along the ventral border of the descending aorta. The esophagus is retracted towards the ventral side and dissected along the ventral margin of the descending aorta until the left mediastinal pleura (Fig. 12.7b). The left mediastinal pleural and lymphoadipose tissues of the left pulmonary ligament are dissected en bloc with the esophagus. Subsequently, all lymphoadipose tissue adjacent to the esophagus is dissected from the pericardium (Fig. 12.7c). The esophagus is pulled up to the right dorsal side. The right mediastinal pleural and lymphoadipose tissues of the right pulmonary ligament are concurrently dissected with the esophagus (Fig. 12.7d). After the subcarinal lymph nodes and both hilar lymph nodes are detached, the esophagus is completely mobilized. A chest tube is inserted into the right pleural cavity.

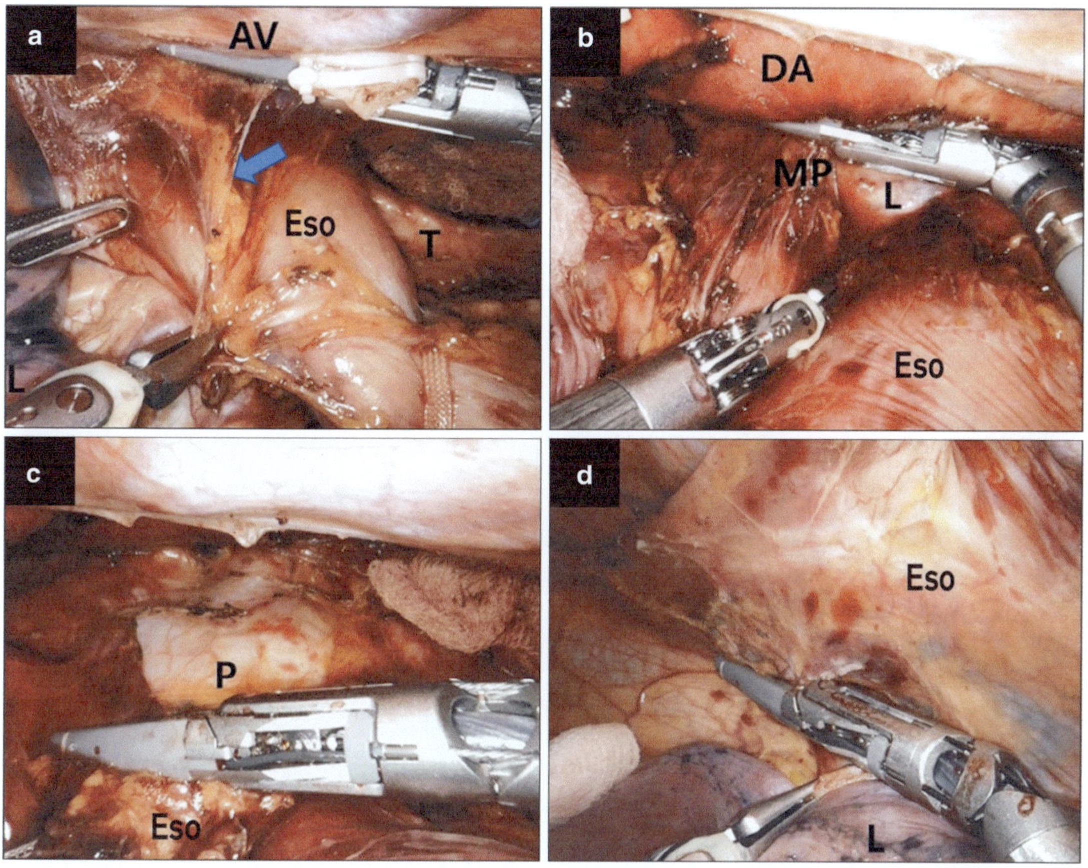

Fig. 12.7 Middle to lower mediastinum dissection. (**a**) Dissection of the thoracic duct. (**b**) Dissection of the dorsal side of the esophagus. (**c**) Dissection of the esophagus from the pericardium. (**d**) Dissection of right mediastinal pleural and lymphoadipose tissue of the right pulmonary ligament. *AV* azygos vein, *Eso* esophagus, *T* trachea, *L* lung, *DA* descending aorta, *MP* left mediastinal pleura, *P* pericardium; blue arrow, thoracic duct

12.5 Bilateral Selective Neck Dissection

The patient is repositioned in the supine position. A soft gel roll is placed at the level of the acromion process to aid neck extension. At our institution, a collar incision is performed by transverse incision within a skin crease of approximately 2 cm or 2 fingerbreadths above the superior edge of the clavicle and sternal notch in a curvilinear fashion. The supraclavicular lymph nodes (Fig. 12.8a) and cervical paraesophageal lymph nodes (Fig. 12.8b) are routinely dissected in all patients (Fig. 12.8c).

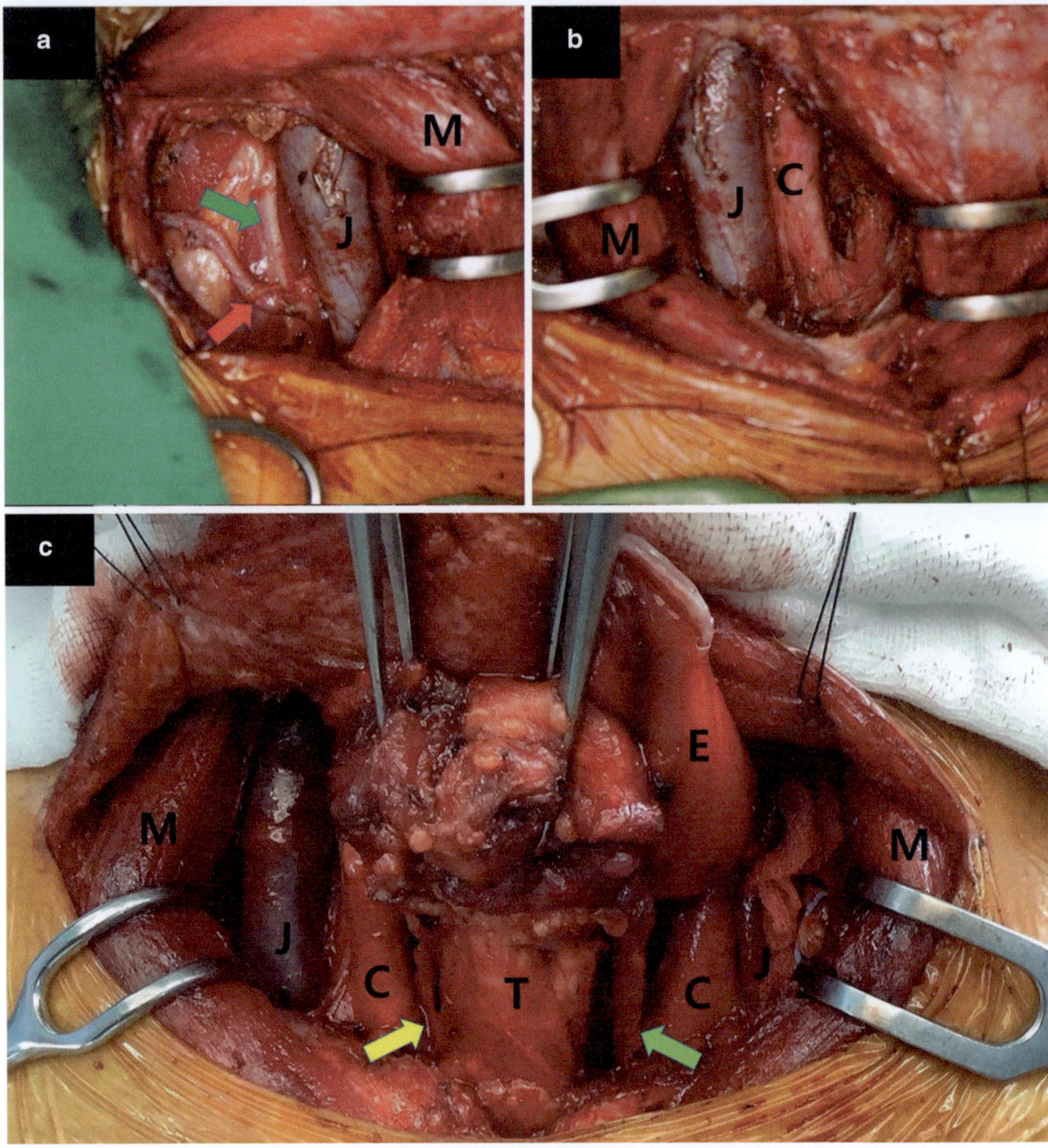

Fig. 12.8 Bilateral selective neck dissection. (**a**) Post-dissection of supraclavicular lymph nodes. (**b**) Post-dissection of cervical paraesophageal lymph nodes. (**c**) Post-bilateral selective neck dissection. *J* jugular vein, *M* sternocleidomastoid, *C* common carotid artery, *E* esophagus, *T* trachea; red arrow, transverse cervical artery; green arrow, phrenic nerve; fluorescent yellow arrow, right recurrent laryngeal nerve; fluorescent green arrow, left recurrent laryngeal nerve

12.6 Gastric Mobilization and Anastomosis

For gastric mobilization, robot-assisted laparoscopy or open laparotomy is performed according to the patient's physical characteristics and preferences. At our institution, both paracardial lymph nodes, lesser curvature lymph nodes, lymph nodes along the left gastric artery, lymph nodes along the common hepatic artery, lymph nodes along the celiac artery, and lymph nodes along the proximal splenic artery are routinely dissected. In most patients, a narrow gastric tube is created along the greater curvature of the stomach using linear staplers, and the staple line is then covered with seromuscular sutures. Pyloroplasty is not performed because we use a narrow gastric tube. The gastric tube is wrapped with a vinyl sheet and pulled up to the neck via a retrosternal route.

At our institution, cervical hand-sewn, double-layered end-to-side esophagogastrostomy is routine. For this procedure, the esophageal wall is divided into a muscular layer and a submucosal layer. The anterior wall of the gastric tube is incised. Interrupted suturing of the muscular layer of the esophagus and the seromuscular layer of the gastric tube is performed, and continuous suturing of the mucosal layers is performed from the posterior side to the anterior side.

12.7 Discussion

McKeown esophagectomy with cervical esophagogastrostomy is the standard surgical approach at our institution. The traditional McKeown approach includes thoracic esophageal dissection via right thoracotomy, gastric mobilization via laparotomy, cervical lymph node dissection, and cervical anastomosis [14]. There are several advantages of the McKeown approach over the Ivor Lewis approach; the former (1) allows more comprehensive lymph node dissection and (2) avoids morbidities associated with intrathoracic anastomosis leakage [15]. However, thoracotomy can lead to increased pulmonary complications, especially in patients with poor pulmonary function. With the goal of decreasing complication rates from such an invasive procedure, various minimally invasive approaches have been developed, including a robot-assisted approach. The advantageous robotic surgery platform provides superior visualization with three-dimensional vision, more degrees of freedom with the endowrist function, and more precise motion with tremor filtering and motion scaling.

It is challenging to completely clear all lymph nodes around the RLN because traction, compression, or thermal injury at any single point leads to nerve palsy. Robot-assisted thoracoscopic surgery has been reported to help reduce these complications. We have previously reported that robot-assisted thoracoscopic surgery has favorable outcomes in terms of left RLN lymph node chain dissections [6, 7]. In a prospective study by Suda et al. [16], robot-assisted thoracoscopic surgery significantly reduced the incidence of vocal cord palsy, hoarseness, and time on the ventilator.

In addition to the application of robot-assisted thoracoscopic surgery, the fascial plane dissection technique helps reduce surgical morbidity. It is based on a specific anatomic concept regarding the relationship between lymphatic structures and the esophagus. This concept is crucial for minimizing the risk of nerve injury during radical lymph node dissection along the RLN. In general, multiple factors affect the occurrence of RLN palsy, including (1) anatomical factors (e.g., the diameter of the nerve and vascular anomaly), (2) patient factors (e.g., a T3 or deeper tumor in the retrotracheal area, a bulky metastatic node along the RLN, a previous history of surgery or irradiation, or high body mass index), and (3) procedural factors (e.g., traction, compression, or thermal injuries to the RLN during dissection). Applying the fascial plane dissection technique in RAMIE eliminates procedural factors, reducing the incidence of RLN palsy to <10%.

In conclusion, the fascial plane dissection technique based on microanatomy could be a reliable method for radical esophagectomy using RAMIE.

Conflict of Interest No potential conflict of interest relevant to this article was reported.

References

1. Van Hillegersberg R, Boone J, Draaisma WA, Broeders IA, Giezeman MJ, Borel Rinkes IH. First experience with robot-assisted thoracoscopic esophagolymphadenectomy for esophageal cancer. Surg Endosc. 2006;20:1435–9.

2. Galvani CA, Gorodner MV, Moser F, et al. Robotically assisted laparoscopic transhiatal esophagectomy. Surg Endosc. 2008;22:188–95.
3. Espat NJ, Jacobsen G, Horgan S, Donahue P. Minimally invasive treatment of esophageal cancer: laparoscopic staging to robotic esophagectomy. Cancer J. 2005;11:10–7.
4. Weksler B, Sharma P, Moudgill N, Chojnacki KA, Rosato EL. Robot-assisted minimally invasive esophagectomy is equivalent to thoracoscopic minimally invasive esophagectomy. Dis Esophagus. 2012;25:403–9.
5. Kim DJ, Park SY, Lee S, Kim HI, Hyung WJ. Feasibility of a robot-assisted thoracoscopic lymphadenectomy along the recurrent laryngeal nerves in radical esophagectomy for esophageal squamous carcinoma. Surg Endosc. 2014;28:1866–73.
6. Park SY, Kim DJ, Yu WS, Jung HS. Robot-assisted thoracoscopic esophagectomy with extensive mediastinal lymphadenectomy: experience with 114 consecutive patients with intrathoracic esophageal cancer. Dis Esophagus. 2016;29:326–32.
7. Park SY, Kim DJ, Kang DR, Haam SJ. Learning curve for robotic esophagectomy and dissection of bilateral recurrent laryngeal nerve nodes for esophageal cancer. Dis Esophagus. 2017;30:1–9.
8. Park SY, Kim DJ, Do YW, Suh J, Lee S. The oncologic outcome of esophageal squamous cell carcinoma patients after robot-assisted thoracoscopic esophagectomy with total mediastinal lymphadenectomy. Ann Thorac Surg. 2017;103:1151–7.
9. Kim DJ, Park SY, Hong MH. Korean experiences of the treatment of esophageal squamous cell carcinoma. In: Ando N, editor. Esophageal squamous cell carcinoma: diagnosis and treatment. 2nd ed. Singapore: Springer Nature; 2020. p. 363–76.
10. Ding X, Zhang J, Li B, et al. A meta-analysis of lymph node metastasis rate for patients with thoracic oesophageal cancer and its implication in delineation of clinical target volume for radiation therapy. Br J Radiol. 2012;85:e1110–9.
11. Wang Y, Zhu L, Xia W, Wang F. Anatomy of lymphatic drainage of the esophagus and lymph node metastasis of thoracic esophageal cancer. Cancer Manag Res. 2018;10:6295–303.
12. Tachimori Y, Nagai Y, Kanamori N, Hokamura N, Igaki H. Pattern of lymph node metastases of esophageal squamous cell carcinoma based on the anatomical lymphatic drainage system. Dis Esophagus. 2011;24:33–8.
13. Park SY, Suh JW, Kim DJ, et al. Near-infrared lymphatic mapping of the recurrent laryngeal nerve nodes in T1 esophageal cancer. Ann Thorac Surg. 2018;105:1613–20.
14. McKeown KC. Trends in oesophageal resection for carcinoma with special reference to total oesophagectomy. Ann R Coll Surg Engl. 1972;51:213–39.
15. D'Amico TA. Mckeown esophagogastrectomy. J Thorac Dis. 2014;6(Suppl 3):S322–4.
16. Suda K, Ishida Y, Kawamura Y, et al. Robot-assisted thoracoscopic lymphadenectomy along the left recurrent laryngeal nerve for esophageal squamous cell carcinoma in the prone position: technical report and short-term outcomes. World J Surg. 2012;36:1608–16.

Totally Robotic Esophagectomy

13

Chang Hyun Kang

Abstract

Totally robotic esophagectomy is performed using a robotic technique without additional thoracoscopy or laparoscopy. However, most robotic esophagectomies are currently performed in a hybrid form combining robotic and other endoscopic techniques. Laparoscopic stomach mobilization and thoracoscopic esophagogastric anastomosis are commonly used methods in robotic esophagectomy. In this paper, totally robotic esophagectomy without thoracoscopic or laparoscopic assistance is presented.

Keywords

Robot surgery · Robot-assisted surgery
Esophagus neoplasms · Esophagectomy
Minimally invasive surgery

13.1 Introduction

Minimally invasive esophagectomy (MIE) has become a standard operative strategy for esophageal cancer. Fewer postoperative complications and early recovery have been documented in many studies [1–9]. Robotic esophagectomy has been performed as an alternative surgical procedure to conventional thoraco-laparoscopic MIE. Robotic esophagectomy also showed early outcomes comparable to those of thoraco-laparoscopic MIE in previous studies [10–18]. However, most of the surgical procedures in those studies were not completely performed using robotic esophagectomy, but were partly performed using laparoscopy, laparotomy, or thoracotomy. Some parts of the operation, including anastomosis and graft formation, have been selectively performed using thoracoscopic or laparoscopic techniques. Therefore, totally robotic esophagectomy (TRE) has been reported in only a few papers. At the author's institution, TRE has been performed since 2008 and it is currently the standard surgical treatment for esophageal cancer. Therefore, this paper presents the surgical technique in detail, along with a brief summary of the surgical outcomes at the Seoul National University Hospital.

C. H. Kang (✉)
Department of Thoracic and Cardiovascular Surgery, Seoul National University Hospital, Seoul National University College of Medicine, Seoul, Republic of Korea
e-mail: chkang@snu.ac.kr

13.2 Abdominal Phase

Ports and Arms

Generally, four robotic ports are made for the abdominal robotic procedure (Fig. 13.1a). Three ports are made using an 8-mm robotic trocar, and the other one is made using a glove port (NELIS,

K. Kim et al. (eds.), *Techniques in Minimally Invasive Thoracic Surgery*,
https://doi.org/10.1007/978-981-19-2472-9_13

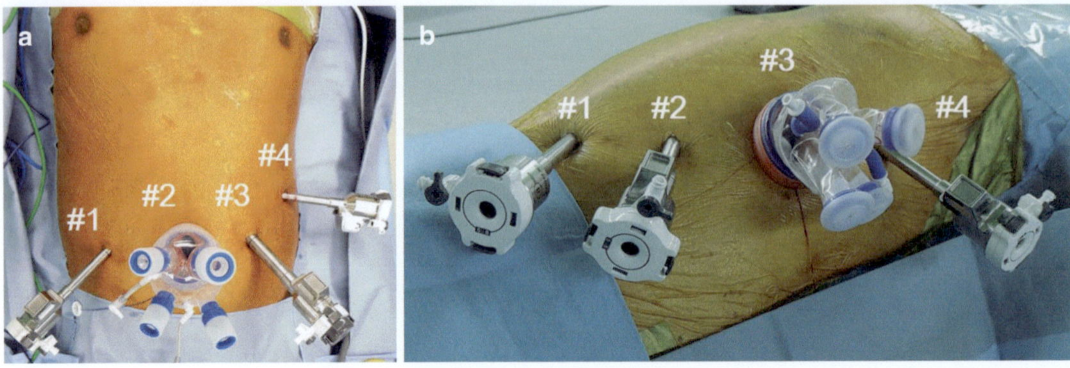

Fig. 13.1 Port placement for the abdominal (**a**) and thoracic (**b**) procedures. The labeled numbers represent the robotic arm number. The detailed location is described in the main text. Robotic staplers are inserted in arm no. 3. Therefore a 12-mm port is necessary for arm no. 3. An assistant surgeon can share the glove port with the robot, and an additional assistant port is not necessary

Table 13.1 The robotic devices used in each arm during abdominal and thoracic procedures

Location	Port no.	Robotic arms
Abdomen	Arm 1	Maryland forceps
	Arm 2	Camera, SureForm stapler[a]
	Arm 3	Scissors, energy device, needle driver, camera[a]
	Arm 4	Force bipolar forceps
Thorax	Arm 1	Maryland forceps
	Arm 2	Scissors, energy device, needle driver, SureForm stapler
	Arm 3	Camera
	Arm 4	Force bipolar forceps

[a]The camera and staplers can be switched with each other during graft stapling

Bucheon, Korea). Usually, a 2-cm port for arm no. 2 is made first in the periumbilical area. This port is mainly used for the robotic camera and the assistant surgeon's work. The port for arm no. 1 is made 10 cm lateral to the periumbilical port. The port for arm no. 3 is made 7.5 cm lateral to the periumbilical port and the port for arm no. 4 is made in the right upward area 7.5 cm lateral to the first right port. The devices used for each trocar are listed in Table 13.1.

Liver Retraction

Liver retraction is usually performed by Prolene suture traction. Prolene (2-0) with a straight needle is passed just below the xiphoid process. The Prolene is sutured to the crus of the diaphragm and again passed out to the right side of the abdominal wall. The suture is tied outside the abdominal wall. The suture can effectively hold up the right lobe of the liver. This simple procedure suffices for the abdominal procedures described below. I do not use a special liver retractor (Fig. 13.2a).

Abdominal Lymph Node Dissection

The dissection of lymph nodes around the celiac axis is crucial for the staging and treatment of esophageal cancer. For complete dissection of the lymph nodes, the lesser omentum is opened widely from the right gastric artery to the hiatus. The dissection usually starts from lymph node station no. 18 (the common hepatic artery lymph

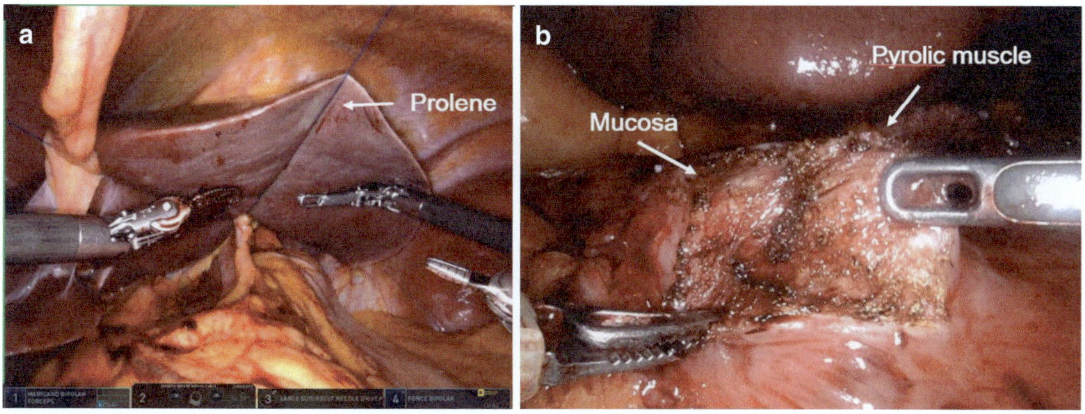

Fig. 13.2 (**a**) Liver retraction can be performed by hanging the liver on prolene string. This procedure makes a liver retractor unnecessary. (**b**) Pyloromyotomy can be performed by fine division of the pyloric muscle. Making the acute angle of the mucosa into a blunt angle between the stomach and duodenum is a key point for successful pyloromyotomy

node) and moves through lymph node station no. 17 (the perigastric lymph node) to lymph node station no. 19 (the splenic artery lymph node). The celiac axis lymph nodes (lymph node station no. 20) can also be removed. However, too deep a dissection along the cisterna chyli increases the risk of chyloperitoneum. If the thoracic duct will be ligated in the chest, the surgeon should remember that the risk of chyloperitoneum increases if radical dissection around the cisterna chyli is performed.

Greater Omentum Division

The greater omentum is generally divided using an energy device (a Harmonic scalpel or Synchroseal is preferred). Usually, a 5-cm distance is maintained from both gastroepiploic arteries. It is important to maintain this distance along the whole length of the greater omentum. In some patients, a direct connection between the right and left gastroepiploic artery does not exist. In that case, the preserved greater omentum can serve as a collateral flow pathway from the right gastroepiploic artery to the fundus. The Kocher maneuver can be performed, and the first and second portions of the duodenum should be completely mobilized. The Kocher maneuver is not necessary in some cases of thoracic anastomosis. However, when the surgeon plans to perform cervical anastomosis, it is safe to perform the Kocher maneuver routinely. It can provide several additional centimeters of conduit.

Pyloromyotomy

Pyloromyotomy can be performed by fine dissection using robotic scissors. Coagulation perpendicular to the pyloric muscle can divide the pyloric ring up to the level of submucosal tissue. The power of monopolar coagulation should be less than two to avoid accidentally damaging the submucosal area. The divided muscle fibers should be partially detached from the submucosal tissue to straighten the angle of the pyloric mucosal fold (Fig. 13.2b). The serosal defect is usually covered by the greater omentum using V-Lock (Medtronic, Dublin, Ireland) continuous sutures.

Graft Formation

When the stomach mobilization procedure is completed, the robotic camera can be changed to port no. 3. After the right gastric artery is divided and clipped, the stomach graft can be made by serial stapling with SureForm staplers. I prefer to

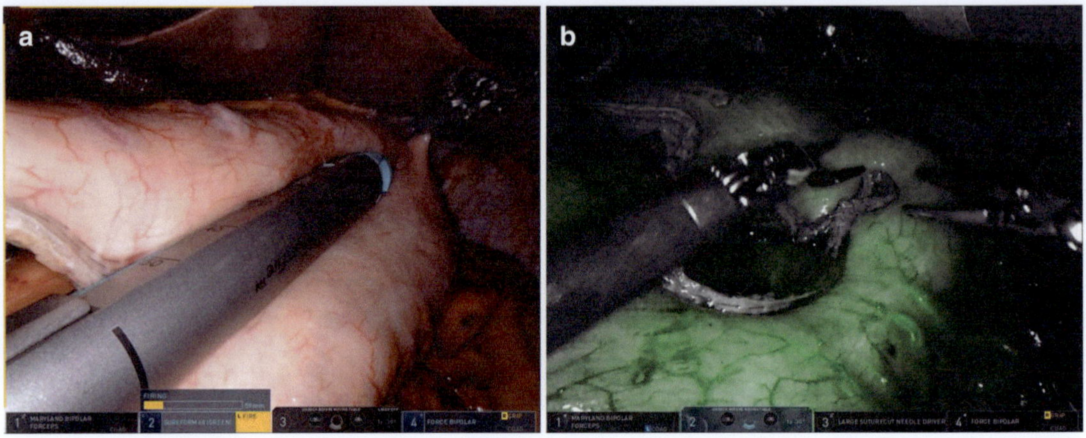

Fig. 13.3 (**a**) Intracorporeal graft formation using a robotic SureForm stapler. The entire graft formation procedure can be completed without additional laparotomy. Robotic staplers increase the degree of freedom of the operating surgeon to determine the shape and the length of the stomach graft. (**b**) Graft blood flow is always checked by indocyanine green infusion after finishing graft formation. Identifying and excluding any ischemic area is important for preventing anastomotic leakage

use 60-mm-sized green staplers to divide the stomach (Fig. 13.3a). Generally, a long graft with a 5-cm width is my preferred method. I routinely check the graft flow using the Firefly system after indocyanine green (ICG) injection (Fig. 13.3b). When selecting an adequate place for anastomosis, I usually check two points: the flow along the marginal artery in the fundus and the serosal uptake of ICG. If the distal fundus does not fulfill those criteria, I usually cut and remove the area with insufficient flow.

13.3 Thoracic Phase

Ports and Arms

Four ports are made for thoracic procedures with the same robotic trocars and glove port used in the abdominal procedure. A port for arm no. 1 is made in the 11th intercostal space at the scapular tip level. A port for arm no. 2 is made 7.5 cm down the right side from port no. 1, and usually at the ninth intercostal space. This port is used for the robotic camera. A port for arm no. 3 is made 7.5 cm to the right, lateral to port no. 2 with a 3-cm size, and a glove port is inserted into this port. This port is shared by the robot and the assistant surgeon. A port for arm no. 4 is made 7.5 cm to the right side of port no. 3 (Fig. 13.1b).

Upper Mediastinum and Dissection of Lymph Nodes Along the Right Recurrent Laryngeal Nerve

As the first step of esophagectomy, the azygos vein is always divided using Hem-o-Lok clips. The right bronchial artery is also ligated during that procedure. After exposing the upper mediastinum, lymph node dissection along the upper thoracic esophagus (lymph node station no. 8U) is performed.

After dividing the mediastinal pleura in the upper mediastinum, lymph node dissection along the right recurrent laryngeal nerve (RLN) can be performed. The proximal part of the right RLN can be identified just below the subclavian artery. Next, the tissues covering the RLN should be completely removed along the right RLN (lymph node station 160RecR in the Japanese Esophageal Society lymph node classification). The limit of the upper end of the dissection is important. The dissection can be performed up to the level of the inferior thyroidal artery and the lower pole of the thyroid gland (Fig. 13.4a).

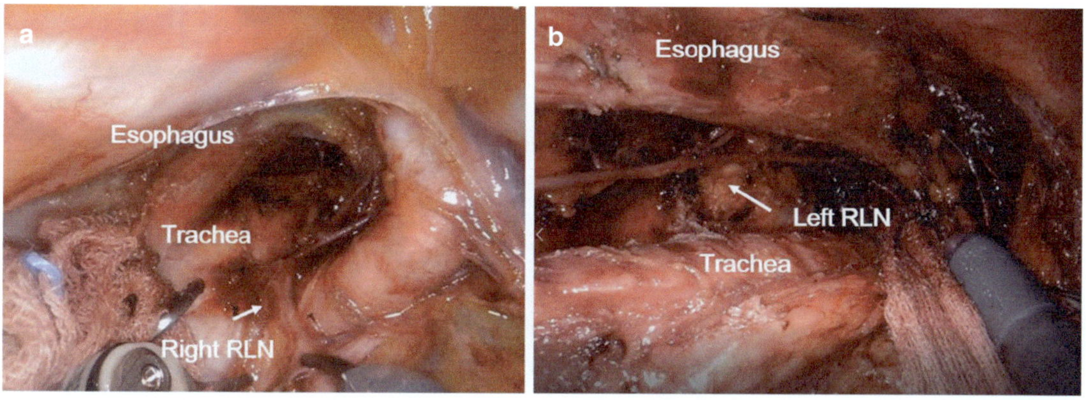

Fig. 13.4 (**a**) Lymph node dissection along the right recurrent laryngeal nerve (RLN). All lymphatic tissues between the right RLN and esophagus can be removed. The dissection can reach the lower pole of the thyroid gland. (**b**) Lymph node dissection along the left RLN by the pre-esophageal approach. The range of dissection is same as on the right side. The dissection can be performed completely in the upper mediastinum and the lower neck

Therefore, dissection of the cervical para-esophageal lymph node can be performed at this stage (lymph node station no. 1R).

Dissection of Lymph Nodes Along the Left Recurrent Laryngeal Nerve

Left RLN dissection can be performed through a retro-esophageal approach or a pre-esophageal approach. I prefer to use the pre-esophageal approach because most lymphatic tissue is located on the medial side of the left RLN. Therefore, retro-esophageal mobilization and exposure of the lateral side of the left RLN are not necessary (Fig. 13.4b). The other advantage of the pre-esophageal approach is better exposure of the lower cervical area. Because the esophagus is located away from the trachea in the pre-esophageal approach, exposure of the lower cervical area is more comfortable than using the retro-esophageal approach. Usually, the left RLN can be identified at the aortic arch level because the lymphatic tissue in this area is thinner than in other areas. Dissection along the left RLN can be performed in the area between the aortic arch and the left main bronchus (lymph node station no. 10L, 106TBL in the Japanese Esophageal Society lymph node classification) and along the left RLN (lymph node station no. 4L and 2L, 106RecL in the Japanese Esophageal Society lymph node classification). The upper limit of the dissection is the same as on the right side (inferior thyroidal artery and lower pole of the thyroid gland), and the left cervical para-esophageal lymph nodes can be removed (lymph node station no. 1L).

Lower Mediastinum and Thoracic Duct Control

Mid and lower-thoracic esophageal dissection is usually performed using an energy device. The vagus nerve is usually divided at the level below the pulmonary branches. The subcarinal (lymph node station no. 7), mid-esophageal (lymph node station no. 8M), lower esophageal (lymph node station no. 8L), both pulmonary ligaments (lymph node station no. 9R and 9L), and diaphragmatic lymph nodes (lymph node station no. 15) are removed at this stage. The thoracic duct is usually not divided and paraaortic tissues are preserved to avoid injuring the thoracic duct. However, if a safe radial margin cannot be achieved with thoracic duct excision or branches of the thoracic duct are injured during dissection, the duct is removed completely from the hiatus to the thoracic inlet level.

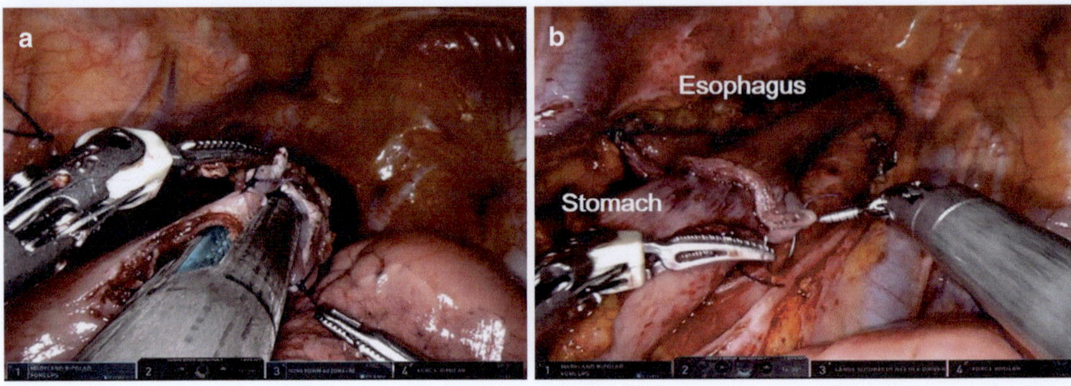

Fig. 13.5 Robotic triangular stapling with SureForm staplers. (**a**) 60-mm SureForm staplers are used to make a large anastomosis circumference. (**b**) The shape of the anastomosis after finishing anterior wall stapling. Wide stretching of the esophageal and gastric walls can be seen. Robotic triangular stapling reduces the anastomosis stricture and prevents postoperative difficulty in swallowing

Gastric Pull-Up and Anastomosis

After finishing the esophageal dissection, the gastric graft can be pulled up and esophagogastric anastomosis can be made at the thoracic inlet level. I prefer to use triangular linear stapling with a robotic SureForm stapler. I usually use 60-mm green staples for this anastomosis (Fig. 13.5a). The goal is to make the diameter of the anastomosis large enough to prevent anastomosis stricture. After finishing the stapling, seromuscular suturing can be performed using V-lock continuous sutures (Fig. 13.5b).

13.4 Outcomes

At the author's institution, TRE was initiated in 2008. However, the main robotic esophagectomy procedure in the early period was a hybrid form with open laparotomy or laparoscopy. The totally robotic approach became the main procedure in 2015, and almost all robotic esophagectomies are now performed using TRE. We have performed 250 TRE cases since 2008. The early outcomes of TRE were favorable, with a 0.4% 30-day mortality and 0.8% 90-day mortality rate. Anastomotic leakage and pulmonary complications occurred in 4.7% and 9.8% of patients, respectively. The overall 5-year survival rate of TRE is 67.0%.

13.5 Discussion

MIE has become one of the standard operations in the treatment of esophageal cancer. In several randomized controlled trials, MIE reduced pulmonary complications, enhanced recovery, and improved quality of life [1–3]. Most centers throughout the world currently perform MIE in significant numbers of patients, and the number of MIEs performed is increasing worldwide [7, 19–21]. The main technique in MIE is a combination of laparoscopic and thoracoscopic techniques. However, there are hybrid forms of MIE using utility thoracotomy and laparotomy for intrathoracic anastomosis and gastric graft formation [22–25]. Currently, there is no clear definition of MIE, and the term "MIE" is used in the literature to describe a wide variety of operations.

The same phenomenon has also occurred in robotic surgery. Technically, robotic esophagectomy should be performed using the robot in both the chest and the abdomen. However, many different types of robotic esophagectomy have been described in the literature. The most common type of robotic esophagectomy is a hybrid form with robotic thoracic procedures and laparoscopic abdominal procedures [3, 26, 27]. Because of the difficulty of thoracoscopic esophagectomy and mediastinal lymph node dissection, the robotic technique has mainly been used for thoracic procedures. However, laparoscopic abdominal procedures have been preferred because of the relative ease of the abdominal procedure. Here, a question can be raised regarding whether the hybrid robotic esophagectomy procedure can truly reflect the advantages of robotic technology.

Robotic technology was developed to improve minimally invasive surgery. Several technological developments have been documented as unique advantages of robotic surgery, including improved camera resolution, a three-dimensional surgical view, full control of the robotic arms by the surgeon, free articulation of the robotic instruments, and many specialized devices dedicated to the robotic system. The benefits of robots can be maximized by fully adapting and maximally utilizing these technological improvements. However, the hybrid form of robotic surgery, which uses laparoscopic and thoracoscopic techniques, cannot fully utilize the robotic system. Therefore, a clear definition of robotic esophagectomy is required and comparative studies between different surgical techniques should be performed. However, it is anticipated that those heterogeneous technical variations will be unified into totally robotic surgery in concordance with advances in robotic technology.

A randomized controlled study comparing robotic and open esophagectomy was recently published [3]. In this trial, robotic esophagectomy improved early postoperative outcomes, with fewer pulmonary complications and improved quality of life. Nonetheless, when compared to thoraco-laparoscopic MIE, the advantages of robotic esophagectomy are unclear. However, several advantages have been suggested in previous studies. The first advantage of robotic esophagectomy is the quality of mediastinal lymph node dissection, especially lymph node dissection around the RLN. The lymph nodes around the RLN are the lymph node stations to which esophageal cancer most commonly metastasizes [28]. They are numbered as 2R, 2L, 4L, and 10L in the American Joint Committee on Cancer system [28], and as 106RecR, 106RecL, and 106Tbl in the Japanese Esophageal Society lymph node map [29]. The dissection of those lymph nodes is technically challenging because of the danger of RLN injury. Nerve injury poses a considerable risk of inducing aspiration pneumonia and deteriorating patients' quality of life. Park et al. [13] compared the quality of mediastinal lymph node dissection, and reported that the number of the dissected lymph nodes along the RLN was higher in robotic esophagectomy than in thoracoscopic esophagectomy. Since then, several other studies have also confirmed the same results, reporting that robotic surgery showed better performance in dissection along the RLN nodes than thoracoscopic surgery [12, 18, 30, 31]. Other researchers reported a reduced incidence of RLN palsy after robotic surgery, which may be another advantage of robotic esophagectomy [32–34]. Zheng et al. [34] also documented a lower incidence of vocal cord palsy in the robotic surgery group in their meta-analysis. The dissection of lymph nodes along both RLNs is the most beneficial aspect of robotic esophagectomy.

In other aspects of esophagectomy, there is not enough evidence to determine whether robotic esophagectomy is better than thoracoscopic or laparoscopic esophagectomy. Na et al. [11] reported similar numbers of dissected lymph nodes in the abdomen compared to laparotomy. However, studies comparing the quality of abdominal procedures in different surgical methods are rare. In terms of the outcomes of anastomosis, the method of robotic anastomosis is quite heterogeneous and the outcomes are not well enough documented for comparison to the thoracoscopic technique. Regarding the respiratory complication rate, the outcomes of robotic surgery and thoracoscopic surgery vary. A meta-analysis paper published by Zheng et al. [34] reported a lower incidence of pulmonary complications in robotic surgery. However, few individual studies have demonstrated a lower incidence of pulmonary complications in robotic surgery. Therefore, those issues should be clarified in future studies.

Long-term survival after MIE has been reported in many studies, and MIE is now generally considered to be comparable to open esophagectomy in terms of long-term survival [2, 35, 36]. However, the long-term survival of patients undergoing robotic esophagectomy has only been reported in a small number of studies in patients with different clinical and pathological stages. Van der Sluis [3] reported comparative outcomes between robotic esophagectomy and open esophagectomy in patients with advanced (stage III and IV) esophageal cancer. The 5-year survival rate of robotic surgery and open surgery was 41% and 40%, respectively, without a significant difference. Park et al. [13] reported long-term outcomes after robotic and thoracoscopic esophagectomy in patients with various stages of the disease. The 5-year overall survival rate of robotic and thoracoscopic esophagectomy was 69% and 59%, respectively; this difference was not statistically significant. According to currently published studies, the long-term survival of patients undergoing robotic esophagectomy is comparable to that of patients undergoing open or thoracoscopic esophagectomy.

Last, learning curve issues should be addressed. Although the outcomes of robotic surgery have been reported for a long time in the literature, many series included early patients who underwent the procedure during the surgeon's learning period. Therefore, the outcomes of robotic surgery in the early period cannot be compared to the outcomes of established centers. The learning curve of a new surgical method can affect the outcomes of esophagectomy at various levels. Park et al. [37] reported that different numbers of cases were necessary for different surgical procedures. This learning curve effect can be shortened by proper proctorship [38]. The learning curve effect should always be considered when interpreting the results of robotic surgery papers. Many centers are still in the early learning period because robotic surgery has been introduced more recently than open esophagectomy or thoraco-laparoscopic MIE.

13.6 Conclusion

In conclusion, robotic esophagectomy is an evolving technique and the outcomes of the operation have improved over the last decades. However, many heterogeneous surgical techniques are currently performed globally and a direct comparison of the outcomes is difficult. TRE is a method that can standardize the robotic surgical technique and maximize the benefits of the robotic surgical system. This article presented the technical aspects of TRE at the author's institution in detail and reviewed the current status of robotic esophagectomy in the literature.

Conflict of Interest Prof. Kang is a consultant doctor of Intuitive Surgical Korea Inc. No potential conflict of interest relevant to this article was reported.

References

1. Biere SS, van Berge Henegouwen MI, Maas KW, et al. Minimally invasive versus open oesophagectomy for patients with oesophageal cancer: a multicentre, open-label, randomised controlled trial. Lancet. 2012;379:1887–92.
2. Mariette C, Markar SR, Dabakuyo-Yonli TS, et al. Hybrid minimally invasive esophagectomy for esophageal cancer. N Engl J Med. 2019;380:152–62.
3. Van der Sluis PC, van der Horst S, May AM, et al. Robot-assisted minimally invasive thoracolaparoscopic esophagectomy versus open transthoracic esophagectomy for resectable esophageal cancer: a randomized controlled trial. Ann Surg. 2019;269:621–30.
4. Briez N, Piessen G, Torres F, Lebuffe G, Triboulet JP, Mariette C. Effects of hybrid minimally invasive oesophagectomy on major postoperative pulmonary complications. Br J Surg. 2012;99:1547–53.
5. Yoshida N, Yamamoto H, Baba H, et al. Can minimally invasive esophagectomy replace open esophagectomy for esophageal cancer? Latest analysis of 24,233 esophagectomies from the Japanese National Clinical Database. Ann Surg. 2020;272:118–24.
6. Booka E, Tsubosa Y, Haneda R, Ishii K. Ability of laparoscopic gastric mobilization to prevent pulmonary complications after open thoracotomy or thoracoscopic esophagectomy for esophageal cancer: a systematic review and meta-analysis. World J Surg. 2020;44:980–9.

7. Takeuchi H, Miyata H, Ozawa S, et al. Comparison of short-term outcomes between open and minimally invasive esophagectomy for esophageal cancer using a nationwide database in Japan. Ann Surg Oncol. 2017;24:1821–7.
8. Luketich JD, Alvelo-Rivera M, Buenaventura PO, et al. Minimally invasive esophagectomy: outcomes in 222 patients. Ann Surg. 2003;238:486–95.
9. Luketich JD, Pennathur A, Awais O, et al. Outcomes after minimally invasive esophagectomy: review of over 1000 patients. Ann Surg. 2012;256:95–103.
10. Van Hillegersberg R, Boone J, Draaisma WA, Broeders IA, Giezeman MJ, Borel Rinkes IH. First experience with robot-assisted thoracoscopic esophagolymphadenectomy for esophageal cancer. Surg Endosc. 2006;20:1435–9.
11. Na KJ, Park S, Park IK, Kim YT, Kang CH. Outcomes after total robotic esophagectomy for esophageal cancer: a propensity-matched comparison with hybrid robotic esophagectomy. J Thorac Dis. 2019;11:5310–20.
12. Chao YK, Hsieh MJ, Liu YH, Liu HP. Lymph node evaluation in robot-assisted versus video-assisted thoracoscopic esophagectomy for esophageal squamous cell carcinoma: a propensity-matched analysis. World J Surg. 2018;42:590–8.
13. Park S, Hwang Y, Lee HJ, Park IK, Kim YT, Kang CH. Comparison of robot-assisted esophagectomy and thoracoscopic esophagectomy in esophageal squamous cell carcinoma. J Thorac Dis. 2016;8:2853–61.
14. Sarkaria IS, Rizk NP. Robotic-assisted minimally invasive esophagectomy: the Ivor Lewis approach. Thorac Surg Clin. 2014;24:211–22.
15. Zhang Y, Han Y, Gan Q, et al. Early outcomes of robot-assisted versus thoracoscopic-assisted Ivor Lewis esophagectomy for esophageal cancer: a propensity score-matched study. Ann Surg Oncol. 2019;26:1284–91.
16. Deng HY, Huang WX, Li G, et al. Comparison of short-term outcomes between robot-assisted minimally invasive esophagectomy and video-assisted minimally invasive esophagectomy in treating middle thoracic esophageal cancer. Dis Esophagus. 2018;31:doy012.
17. Deng HY, Luo J, Li SX, et al. Does robot-assisted minimally invasive esophagectomy really have the advantage of lymphadenectomy over video-assisted minimally invasive esophagectomy in treating esophageal squamous cell carcinoma? A propensity score-matched analysis based on short-term outcomes. Dis Esophagus. 2019;32:doy110.
18. Yang Y, Zhang X, Li B, et al. Short- and mid-term outcomes of robotic versus thoraco-laparoscopic McKeown esophagectomy for squamous cell esophageal cancer: a propensity score-matched study. Dis Esophagus. 2020;33:doz080.
19. Sihag S, Kosinski AS, Gaissert HA, Wright CD, Schipper PH. Minimally invasive versus open esophagectomy for esophageal cancer: a comparison of early surgical outcomes from the Society of Thoracic Surgeons National Database. Ann Thorac Surg. 2016;101:1281–9.
20. Seesing MF, Gisbertz SS, Goense L, et al. A propensity score matched analysis of open versus minimally invasive transthoracic esophagectomy in the Netherlands. Ann Surg. 2017;266:839–46.
21. Mamidanna R, Bottle A, Aylin P, Faiz O, Hanna GB. Short-term outcomes following open versus minimally invasive esophagectomy for cancer in England: a population-based national study. Ann Surg. 2012;255:197–203.
22. Bonavina L, Scolari F, Aiolfi A, et al. Early outcome of thoracoscopic and hybrid esophagectomy: propensity-matched comparative analysis. Surgery. 2016;159:1073–81.
23. Ichikawa H, Miyata G, Miyazaki S, et al. Esophagectomy using a thoracoscopic approach with an open laparotomic or hand-assisted laparoscopic abdominal stage for esophageal cancer: analysis of survival and prognostic factors in 315 patients. Ann Surg. 2013;257:873–85.
24. Fumagalli U, Baiocchi GL, Celotti A, et al. Incidence and treatment of mediastinal leakage after esophagectomy: insights from the multicenter study on mediastinal leaks. World J Gastroenterol. 2019;25:356–66.
25. Mu JW, Gao SG, Xue Q, et al. Updated experiences with minimally invasive McKeown esophagectomy for esophageal cancer. World J Gastroenterol. 2015;21:12873–81.
26. Zhang X, Su Y, Yang Y, et al. Robot assisted esophagectomy for esophageal squamous cell carcinoma. J Thorac Dis. 2018;10:3767–75.
27. Yun JK, Chong BK, Kim HJ, et al. Comparative outcomes of robot-assisted minimally invasive versus open esophagectomy in patients with esophageal squamous cell carcinoma: a propensity score-weighted analysis. Dis Esophagus. 2020;33:doz071.
28. Akutsu Y, Kato K, Igaki H, et al. The prevalence of overall and initial lymph node metastases in clinical T1N0 thoracic esophageal cancer: from the results of JCOG0502, a prospective multicenter study. Ann Surg. 2016;264:1009–15.
29. Japan Esophageal Society. Japanese Classification of Esophageal Cancer, 11th edition: part II and III. Esophagus. 2017;14:37–65.
30. Xu Y, Li XK, Cong ZZ, et al. Long-term outcomes of robotic-assisted versus thoraco-laparoscopic McKeown esophagectomy for esophageal cancer: a propensity score-matched study. Dis Esophagus. 2020;34(9):doaa114. https://doi.org/10.1093/dote/doaa114.
31. Duan X, Yue J, Chen C, et al. Lymph node dissection around left recurrent laryngeal nerve: robot-assisted vs. video-assisted McKeown esophagectomy for esophageal squamous cell carcinoma. Surg Endosc. 2020;35(11):6108–16. https://doi.org/10.1007/s00464-020-08105-2.
32. Suda K, Ishida Y, Kawamura Y, et al. Robot-assisted thoracoscopic lymphadenectomy along the left recurrent laryngeal nerve for esophageal squamous cell

carcinoma in the prone position: technical report and short-term outcomes. World J Surg. 2012;36:1608–16.
33. Oshikiri T, Goto H, Horikawa M, et al. Incidence of recurrent laryngeal nerve palsy in robot-assisted versus conventional minimally invasive McKeown esophagectomy in prone position: a propensity score-matched study. Ann Surg Oncol. 2021;28(12):7249–57. https://doi.org/10.1245/s10434-021-10123-w.
34. Zheng C, Li XK, Zhang C, et al. Comparison of short-term clinical outcomes between robot-assisted minimally invasive esophagectomy and video-assisted minimally invasive esophagectomy: a systematic review and meta-analysis. J Thorac Dis. 2021;13:708–19.
35. Straatman J, van der Wielen N, Cuesta MA, et al. Minimally invasive versus open esophageal resection: three-year follow-up of the previously reported randomized controlled trial: the TIME trial. Ann Surg. 2017;266:232–6.
36. Gottlieb-Vedi E, Kauppila JH, Malietzis G, Nilsson M, Markar SR, Lagergren J. Long-term survival in esophageal cancer after minimally invasive compared to open esophagectomy: a systematic review and meta-analysis. Ann Surg. 2019;270:1005–17.
37. Park S, Hyun K, Lee HJ, Park IK, Kim YT, Kang CH. A study of the learning curve for robotic oesophagectomy for oesophageal cancer. Eur J Cardiothorac Surg. 2018;53:862–70.
38. Van der Sluis PC, Ruurda JP, van der Horst S, Goense L, van Hillegersberg R. Learning curve for robot-assisted minimally invasive thoracoscopic esophagectomy: results from 312 cases. Ann Thorac Surg. 2018;106:264–71.

Management of Anastomotic Leakage

14

Jae Hyun Jeon

Abstract

The treatment options for post-esophagectomy leakage remain a matter of debate and lack standardization even at individual facilities. The principles of managing postoperative leakage depend on the location of the anastomotic leakage, defect size, the time elapsed until treatment after the occurrence of leakage, and the patient's physiological condition. Strategies include conservative management (involving strict restrictions on oral intake, systemic antibiotics, and appropriate drainage), endoscopic techniques, and surgical exploration. Although there is no consensus guideline, there has been a progressive shift in treatment strategies from an aggressive surgical approach toward more conservative management and endoscopic interventions. This review presents an overview of effective therapeutic options for postoperative leakage after esophagectomy.

Keywords

Esophagectomy · Leakage · Endoscopic management

J. H. Jeon (✉)
Department of Thoracic and Cardiovascular Surgery, Seoul National University Bundang Hospital, Seoul National University College of Medicine, Seongnam, Gyeonggi-Do, Republic of Korea
e-mail: jhjeon@snubh.org

14.1 Introduction

Radical esophagectomy provides the highest likelihood of a cure for patients who have potentially resectable esophageal cancer. Although advances in perioperative management and surgical techniques have led to reductions in postoperative morbidity and mortality, postoperative leakage is among the most dreaded complications and continues to be a cause of postoperative mortality. The reported incidence of postoperative leakage after esophagectomy varies from 11.4 to 21.2%, with an associated mortality rates as high as 7.2–35% [1–3]. The clinical manifestations of postoperative leakage range from clinically silent cases to fulminant sepsis and life-threatening conditions. A study conducted in 2012 using nationwide data from Sweden reported a mortality rate of 18.2% for postoperative anastomotic leakage, reflecting a threefold higher mortality rate than observed in patients who did not experience this complication [4].

The treatment options for postoperative anastomotic leakage remain a matter of debate and lack standardization even at individual facilities [5]. The principles of managing anastomotic leakage depend on the location of anastomotic leakage, defect size, the time elapsed until treatment after the occurrence of leakage, and the patient's physiological condition. Strategies include conservative management (involving strict restrictions on oral intake, sys-

K. Kim et al. (eds.), *Techniques in Minimally Invasive Thoracic Surgery*,
https://doi.org/10.1007/978-981-19-2472-9_14

temic antibiotics, and appropriate drainage), endoscopic techniques, and surgical exploration. Although there is no consensus guideline, there has been a progressive shift in treatment strategies from an aggressive surgical approach toward more conservative management and endoscopic interventions.

This review presents an overview of effective therapeutic options for postoperative anastomotic leakage.

14.2 Conservative Management

The basic principles of conservative treatment include gastrointestinal decompression, adequate drainage, infection control, and nutritional support. It is necessary to keep patients on strict nothing-by-mouth management together with parenteral or enteral nutrition (jejunostomy) for 1–3 weeks (median). Broad-spectrum antibiotics covering anaerobic, Gram-negative, and Gram-positive should be administered. It is important to perform adequate drainage (through surgery or by using a percutaneous catheter) for collections of contaminated fluid in the pericardium, pleural space, and mediastinum, in addition to lung abscesses, to prevent further propagation of infection. Although an external drain can be used to manage leakage, it is common to use a nasogastric (NG) tube for simultaneous decompression of the conduit to minimize continuing contamination from leakage at the anastomosis site.

14.3 Endoscopic Stent

The endoscopic stent technique involves placing a prosthesis in the esophageal lumen to cover the anastomotic defect until the tissue heals. With the development and improvement of biomaterials, endoscopic stent placement became the treatment of choice for symptomatic leakage in patients with no signs of sepsis or severe conduit ischemia [6]. Over the years, various materials including self-expanding plastic stents (SEPS) and metal stents (SEMS) have been evaluated for the management of post-esophagectomy leakage. These stents usually remain in place for 2–4 weeks prior to removal, and the leakage site is reevaluated endoscopically to determine whether closure has taken place. Boeckel et al. reported the efficacy and safety of various types of stents in a systemic review [7]. Eighty-five percent of patients showed clinical success, with no significant difference between stent types (84% for SEPS, 85% for fully covered SEMS, and 86% for partially covered SEMS, $p = 0.97$). The longest duration of stent placement was found in patients who received SEPS (8 weeks), followed by those who received fully covered SEMS and partially covered SEMS. With regard to tissue migration and tissue overgrowth, which can be considered the two principal complications, fully covered SEMS ensures a more favorable balance. A higher risk of tissue overgrowth is found in partially covered SEMS with non-coated terminal regions, while a higher migration risk is observed in SEPS. The risk of failure is typically high in procedures for proximal cervical leakage, primarily as a result of the difficulty of performing fixation in the remaining esophagus and the resultant propensity for stent migration. Furthermore, placing a stent in close proximity to the esophageal sphincter can result in airway compromise, globus sensation, pain, and aspiration pneumonia. Other complications (e.g., stent-related bleeding and perforation) can be lethal, which has prompted research attempting to identify preferable modalities [8].

14.4 Endoscopic Vacuum Therapy

Vacuum-assisted closure (VAC) can serve as an alternative option instead of conventional wound management. Negative pressure has demonstrated its efficacy in the treatment of external wounds, as exemplified by pressure sores. VAC therapy primarily induces healing by reducing localized tissue edema, removing purulent discharge, increasing local perfusion, and promoting the formulation of granulation tissue [9]. Endoscopic vacuum therapy (EVT) is expected to yield similar results when applied to manage post-esophagectomy leakage [10]. In EVT, a polyurethane sponge connected to a NG tube is endoscopically placed in the lumen or abscess cavity. The application of a continuous negative pressure system results in decreased interstitial edema and bacterial contamination, improved tissue perfusion, and rapid formation of healthy granulation tissue, leading to a gradual decrease in the size of the cavity (Figs. 14.1 and 14.2) and, eventually, complete closure [11].

Herein, we describe the technique in detail and present our initial findings [12]. EVT is initiated on the day that leakage is diagnosed endoscopically or, if necessary, 1 day later. Prior to the procedure, an appropriately sized polyurethane sponge (KCI, San Antonio, TX, USA) is determined according to the defect size. An NG tube (Levin, 16-Fr; Insung Medical, Seoul, Korea) is inserted into a single nostril following the application of a lubricating gel, and grasping forceps are then used to extract the tube through the oral cavity. To maintain the negative pressure at the location where the polyurethane sponge wraps the NG tube, the tip of the NG tube is cut to the last side hole, resulting in the formation of a large hole at the end of the NG tube. The size-adjusted

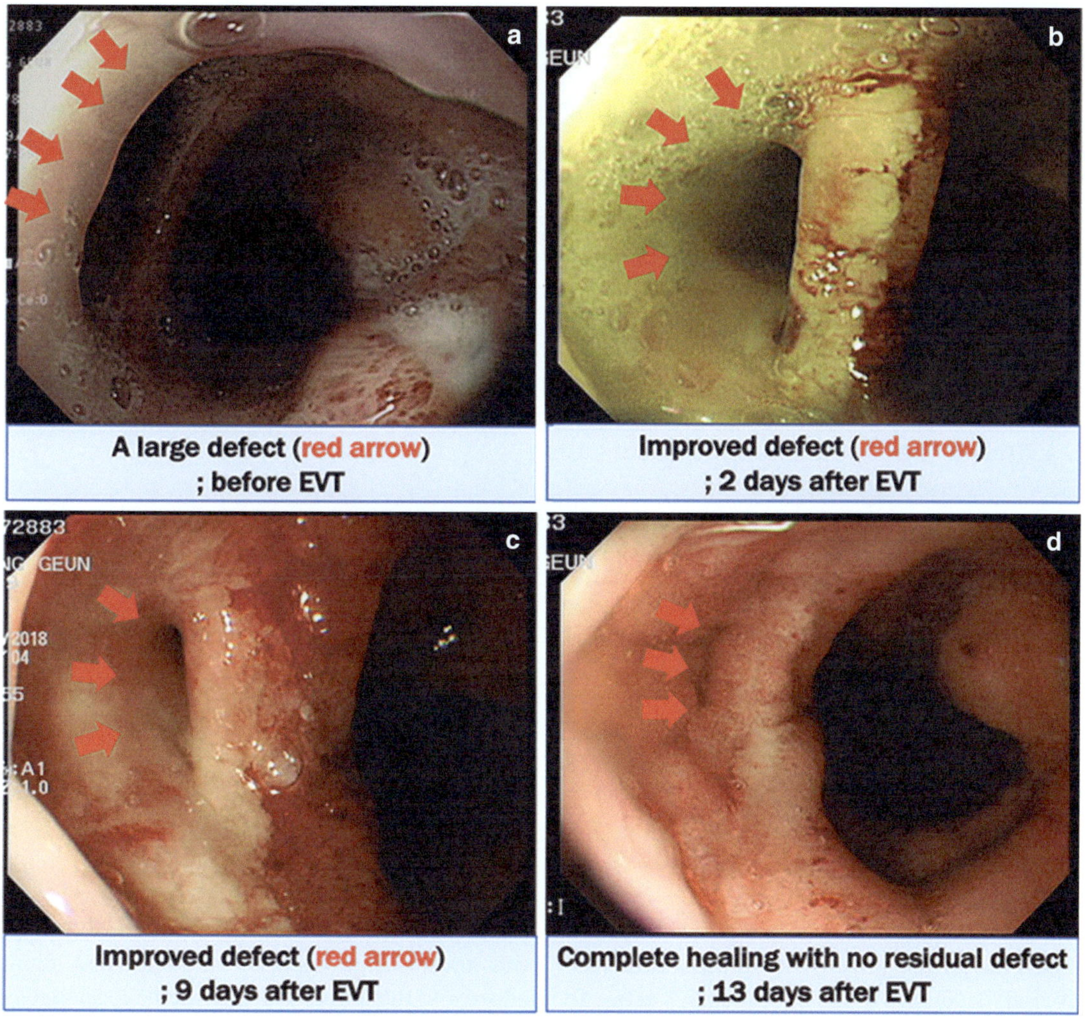

Fig. 14.1 A large anastomotic defect was completely healed during endoscopic vacuum therapy (EVT). (**a**) Initial diagnosis, with a large defect around the anastomosis. (**b**–**d**) During EVT, with regular changes of the sponge at intervals of 3–5 days, complete healing was achieved. The arrow indicates anastomotic leakage

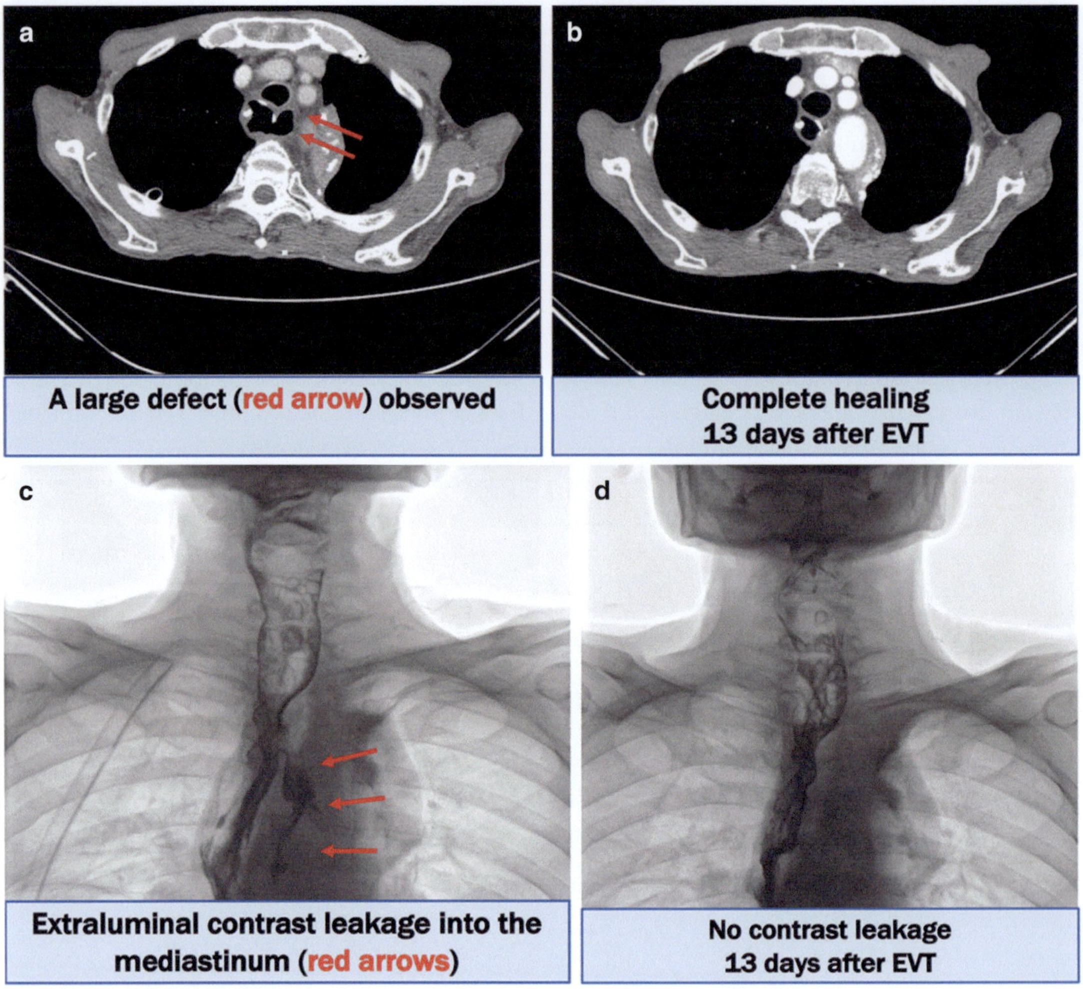

Fig. 14.2 Large anastomotic defect was completely healed during endoscopic vacuum therapy (EVT). The arrow indicates anastomotic leakage. (**a**) A large defect was observed on chest computed tomography (chest CT). (**b**) Complete healing was observed 13 days after EVT (chest CT). (**c**) Extraluminal contrast leakage into the mediastinum on esophagography. (**d**) Complete healing was observed 13 days after EVT (esophagography)

polyurethane sponge is then sutured to the tip of the NG tube at three points using 3-0 nylon. Grasping the polyurethane sponge, the endoscope is inserted into the esophagus (Fig. 14.3). The polyurethane sponge is then moved into the intraluminal or cavitary space (Fig. 14.4). If possible, the sponge is positioned in the wound cavity, and the polyurethane sponge is shaped to match the precise dimensions of the wound (15–30 mm) according to the endoscopist's estimate. If there are multiple cavities that are too small for endoscopic access, it is possible to place the sponge in the esophageal lumen. As proposed by Loske et al., it is necessary for the sponge to be larger than the intracavitary counterpart (roughly 1.5–2 cm in diameter and 4–5 cm in length), since the sponge must cover the defect [13]. When an electronic vacuum device is connected (KCI V.A.C. Freedom®, KCI USA Inc., San Antonio, TX, USA; settings: – 125 mmHg, continuous, and high intensity), the open-pore foam adheres to the tissue. The polyurethane sponge is changed at intervals of 3–4 days. When the sponge is changed, the organs surrounding the

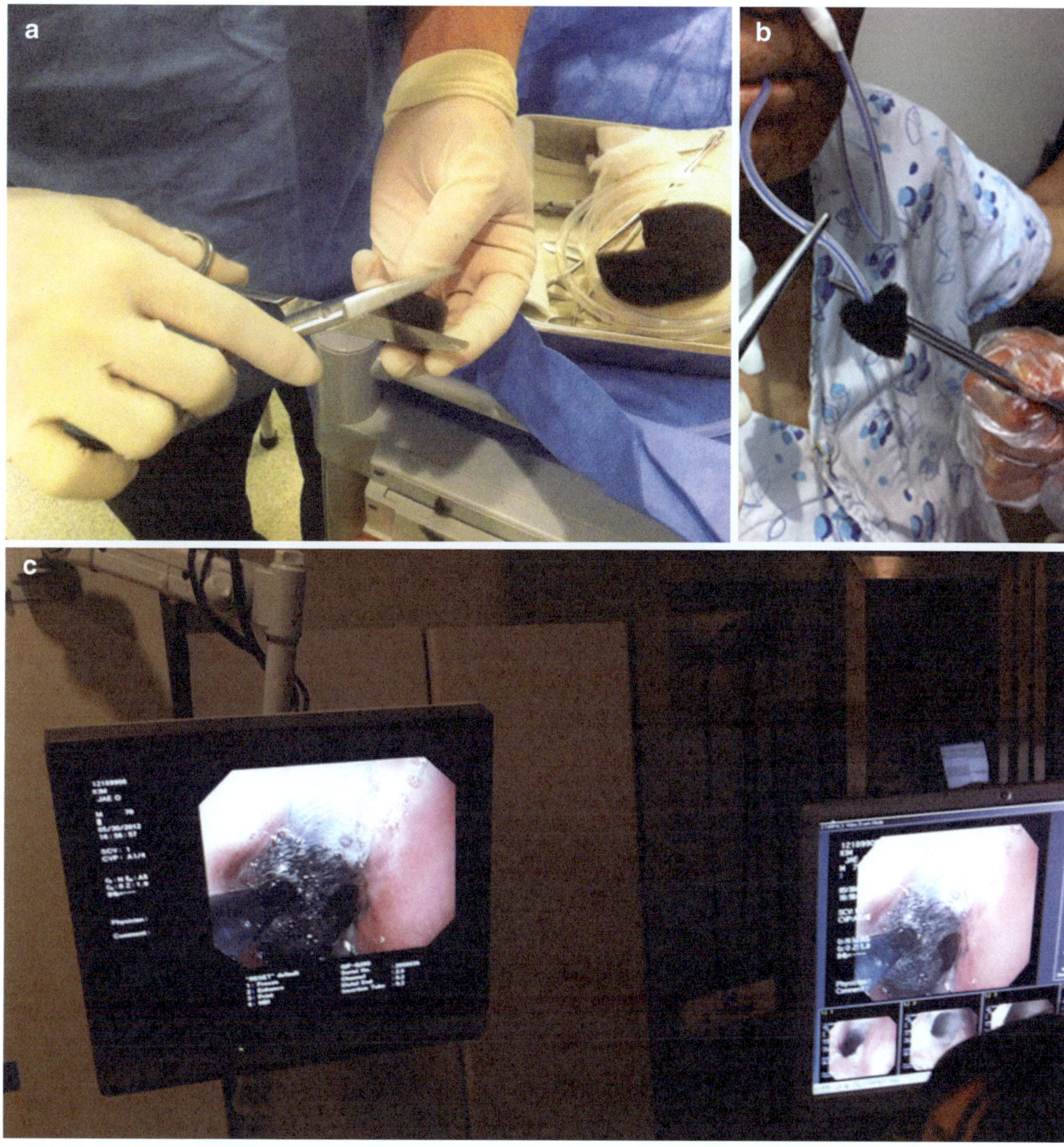

Fig. 14.3 (**a**) Size-adjusted sponge (pore size, 400–600 mm). (**b**) Insertion of a nasogastric tube into a nostril after application of a lubricating gel, followed by extraction through the oral cavity with forceps. (**c**) The sponge was grasped using grasping forceps and introduced into the necrotic cavities using a standard forward-view endoscope

leakage site should be carefully evaluated and periodic endoscopic inspections should be performed to evaluate the granulation tissue growth pattern during EVT in order to avoid EVT-related complications. Between May 2012 and April 2018, 22 patients received treatment at our hospital with intracavitary or intraluminal EVT to manage postoperative leakage [12]. In 19 of these patients (86.4%), it was possible to achieve complete closure. The median duration of EVT application was 14 days (range 2–103 days), and the median number of EVT systems used was three

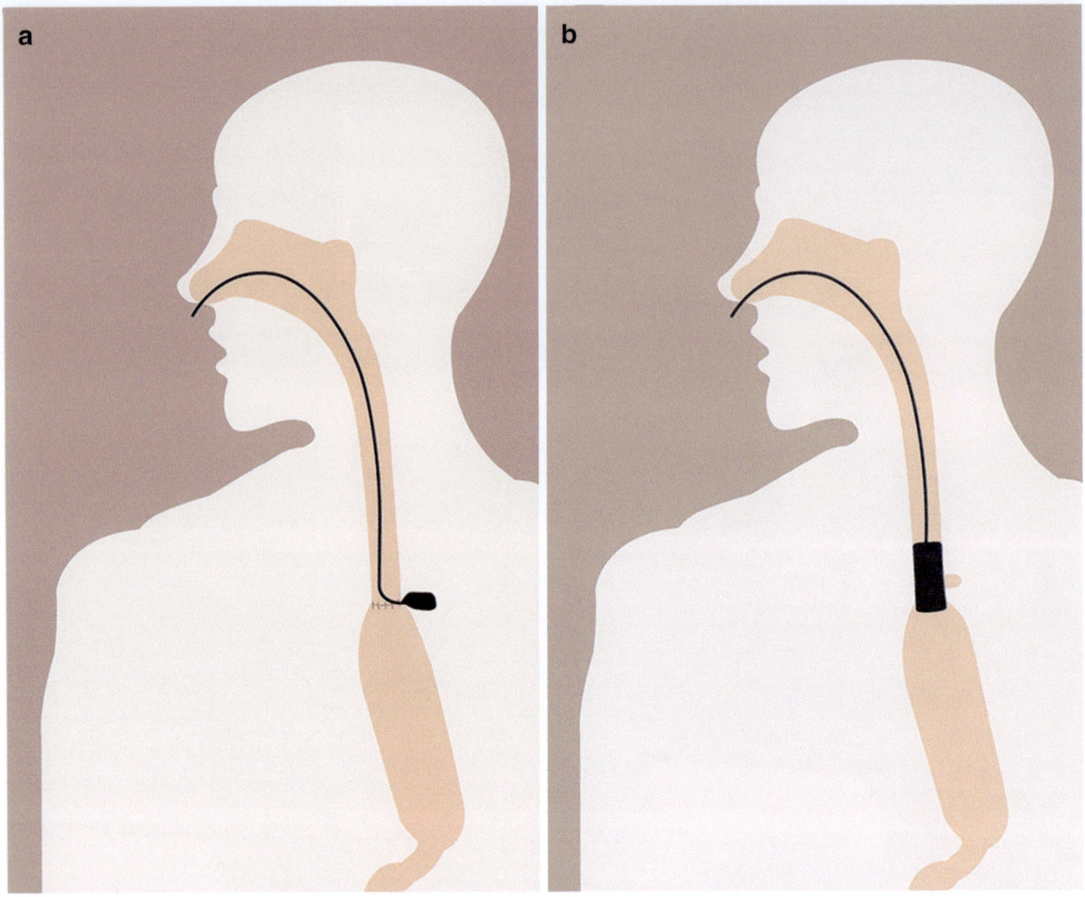

Fig. 14.4 Illustrations of endoscopic vacuum therapy (EVT) with (**a**) intracavitary and (**b**) intraluminal sponge placement

(range 1–14 systems). In the 19 cases of successful management using EVT, oral feeding became possible at a median of 15 days following the first day of treatment. No instances of postoperative leakage-related mortality were observed.

A meta-analysis of 18 published studies reported high technical and clinical success rates (97.1% and 89.4%, respectively) and low rates of adverse events and all-cause mortality (13.6% and 7.1%, respectively) using EVT [14]. In recent years, EVT has developed into a valuable alternative for postoperative leakage after esophagectomy, and innovative drainage materials have been developed accordingly. Newly developed open-pore materials (e.g., a film-coated sponge and a small-caliber, open-pore film drain) show less adherence and decrease the likelihood of severe bleeding. A certified and commercially available drainage system based on the overtube principle has been distributed (Eso-SPONGE®, B. Braun Melsungen AG, Melsungen, Germany) [15]. However, approved medical devices and novel open-pore materials to treat esophageal leakage are still not available in Asia. We may hope that partners in industry will soon take an interest in and promote this therapy, which would make it possible to use standardized and optimized materials instead of ad-hoc, self-made materials. This would also enable comparative studies.

14.5 Surgical Treatment

The surgical indications for postoperative leakage are usually patient-tailored, taking into consideration the location of anastomotic leakage, the defect size, the time that has elapsed until treatment after leak occurrence, and the patient's physiological condition. Several studies comparing non-operative treatments and surgical intervention have demonstrated no statistically significant differences in the time to leak closure according to whether patients underwent surgical exploration or received conservative management [16, 17]. Surgical treatment is generally considered (1) for patients with "early leakages," which are usually not contained, resulting in generalized inflammation of the pleural cavity and severe sepsis; (2) for cases of leakage after the failure of endoscopic and/or conservative treatment; and (3) for severely septic patients [18]. Surgical options include primary repair of the defect with debridement and drainage, as well as tacking down the conduit with either immediate or delayed reconstruction. The viability of the gastric tube mucosa is an important factor when deciding upon the type of surgery to perform, and an endoscopic evaluation before surgical exploration is mandatory. Diffuse ischemia and necrosis of the gastric conduit will often not be salvageable and may require anastomosis takedown and the temporary creation of a cervical esophagostomy. Once full recovery takes place, it is possible to restore the gastrointestinal continuity by interposing tissue from the colon or jejunum. If the defect is local, without ischemia or necrosis, it is usually possible to preserve the gastric conduit and perform primary repair of the defect. If local ischemia of the gastric fundus tip occurs, the necrotic tissue can be resected, with immediate re-anastomosis.

14.6 Conclusion

The diversity of the presentation and severity of leakage, along with the multiplicity of available therapeutic methods, are challenges for optimal management. Once postoperative leakage after esophagectomy is diagnosed or strongly suspected, patient-tailored strategies should be implemented depending on the location of anastomotic leakage, the defect size, the time elapsed since the leak occurred, and the patient's physiological status. The management of postoperative leakage after esophagectomy has shifted from aggressive surgical interventions to conservative management, and more recently, endoscopic interventions (SEMS, EVT, etc.) have been utilized with increasing frequency. According to the extant data, EVT is feasible, effective, and safe, with favorable clinical outcomes in the short-term and long-term management of post-esophagectomy leakage.

Acknowledgments and Disclosures The author declares that there is no conflict of interest relevant to this paper.

References

1. van Workum F, van der Maas J, van den Wildenberg FJ, Polat F, Kouwenhoven EA, van Det MJ, et al. Improved functional results after minimally invasive esophagectomy: intrathoracic versus cervical anastomosis. Ann Thorac Surg. 2017;103:267–73.
2. Schmidt HM, Gisbertz SS, Moons J, Rouvelas I, Kauppi J, Brown A, et al. Defining benchmarks for transthoracic esophagectomy: a multicenter analysis of total minimally invasive esophagectomy in low risk patients. Ann Surg. 2017;266:814–21.
3. Low DE, Kuppusamy MK, Alderson D, Cecconello I, Chang AC, Darling G, et al. Benchmarking complications associated with esophagectomy. Ann Surg. 2019;269:291–8.
4. Rutegård M, Lagergren P, Rouvelas I, Lagergren J. Intrathoracic anastomotic leakage and mortality after esophageal cancer resection: a population-based study. Ann Surg Oncol. 2012;19:99–103.
5. Schaheen L, Blackmon SH, Nason KS. Optimal approach to the management of intrathoracic esophageal leak following esophagectomy: a systematic review. Am J Surg. 2014;208:536–43.
6. Ong GKB, Freeman RK. Endoscopic management of esophageal leaks. J Thorac Dis. 2017;9:S135–45.
7. van Boeckel PG, Sijbring A, Vleggaar FP, Siersema PD. Systematic review: temporary stent placement for benign rupture or anastomotic leak of the oesophagus. Aliment Pharmacol Ther. 2011;33:1292–301.
8. Hindy P, Hong J, Lam-Tsai Y, Gress F. A comprehensive review of esophageal stents. Gastroenterol Hepatol. 2012;8:526–34.
9. Argenta LC, Morykwas MJ. Vacuum-assisted closure: a new method for wound control and treatment: clinical experience. Ann Plast Surg. 1997;38:563–76.
10. Loske G, Schorsch T, Müller C. Endoscopic vacuum sponge therapy for esophageal defects. Surg Endosc. 2010;24:2531–5.
11. Kuehn F, Schiffmann L, Rau BM, Klar E. Surgical endoscopic vacuum therapy for anastomotic leakage

and perforation of the upper gastrointestinal tract. J Gastrointest Surg. 2012;16:2145–50.
12. Jeon JH, Jang HJ, Han JE, Park YS, Seong YW, Cho S, et al. Endoscopic vacuum therapy in the management of postoperative leakage after esophagectomy. World J Surg. 2020;44:179–85.
13. Loske G, Schorsch T, Muller C. Intraluminal and intracavitary vacuum therapy for esophageal leakage: a new endoscopic minimally invasive approach. Endoscopy. 2011;43:540–4.
14. Aziz M, Haghbin H, Sharma S, Weissman S, Saleem S, Lee-Smith W, et al. Safety and effectiveness of endoluminal vacuum-assisted closure for esophageal defects: systematic review and meta-analysis. Endosc Int Open. 2021;9:E1371–80.
15. Loske G, Muller CT. Tips and tricks for endoscopic negative pressure therapy. Chirurg. 2019;90:7–14.
16. Lee DH, Kim HR, Kim SR, Kim YH, Kim DK, Park SI. Comparison of clinical outcomes after conservative and surgical treatment of isolated anastomotic leaks after esophagectomy for esophageal cancer. Dis Esophagus. 2013;26:609–15.
17. Guo J, Chu X, Liu Y, Zhou N, Ma Y, Liang C. Choice of therapeutic strategies in intrathoracic anastomotic leak following esophagectomy. World J Surg Oncol. 2014;12:402.
18. Famiglietti A, Lazar JF, Henderson H, Hamm M, Malouf S, Margolis M, et al. Management of anastomotic leaks after esophagectomy and gastric pull-up. J Thorac Dis. 2020;12:1022–30.

Part III

Others

Video-Assisted Thoracoscopic Surgery Thymectomy: Transpleural Approach

15

In Kyu Park

Abstract

There are several types of minimally invasive approaches for thymectomy, of which the transpleural approach by video-assisted thoracoscopic surgery is particularly useful. In this approach, thymectomy is performed from either side of the thoracic cage. Thoracic surgeons should be familiar with the principles of the procedure, the anatomy of the region, and surgical strategies for successful thymectomy. The details of transpleural thymectomy are discussed herein.

Keywords

Thymectomy · Video-assisted thoracic surgery · Myasthenia gravis · Thymus neoplasms

15.1 Introduction

Thymectomy is performed for the treatment of a wide range of thymic diseases, such as benign tumors, malignant tumors, and myasthenia gravis. The extent of thymectomy is tailored according to the disease condition. Total thymectomy is recommended for malignant tumors [1]. Partial thymectomy can be considered for benign tumors and early-stage thymoma in highly selected patients [2]. Extended thymectomy, which includes the radical removal of ectopic thymic tissue, is recommended in myasthenia gravis [3].

The lateral approach using video-assisted thoracoscopic surgery (VATS) is a useful method for thymectomy. Surgeons can choose a unilateral approach on either side or a bilateral approach to accomplish the surgical and oncologic goals. Additional cervical incision, upper partial sternotomy, or subxiphoid incision can be helpful in specific situations.

There is a global consensus on the principles that apply to surgical resection in general, as well as minimally invasive surgery for thymic neoplasms [4, 5]. Surgeons should familiarize themselves with these guidelines prior to performing VATS thymectomy.

15.2 Procedures and Techniques

Anesthesia

General anesthesia with double-lumen endotracheal intubation is used in general. Selective ventilation with CO_2 insufflation provides an excellent operative view and space. Single-lumen endotracheal tube intubation and controlled ventilation can also be used in combination with CO_2 insuf-

I. K. Park (✉)
Department of Thoracic and Cardiovascular Surgery, Seoul National University Hospital, Seoul National University College of Medicine, Seoul, Republic of Korea
e-mail: ikpark@snu.ac.kr

K. Kim et al. (eds.), *Techniques in Minimally Invasive Thoracic Surgery*,
https://doi.org/10.1007/978-981-19-2472-9_15

flation. Nonintubated general anesthesia with or without a laryngeal mask under deep sedation can be applied for simple procedures [6].

Position of the Patient and Surgery Team

The most popular patient position is the semi-supine position up to 30°. The patient is placed in the supine position with a roll placed under the ipsilateral chest [7, 8]. The ipsilateral arm is abducted or dropped below the chest to expose the axillary area. The contralateral arm is also positioned in the same way if the bilateral approach has been planned. The arms should not interfere with the course of the instruments, especially those inserted through the axillary area. Care should be taken to not overextend the shoulder.

The operator and the assistant stand on the ipsilateral side of the patients, while the scrub nurse stands on the contralateral side (Fig. 15.1).

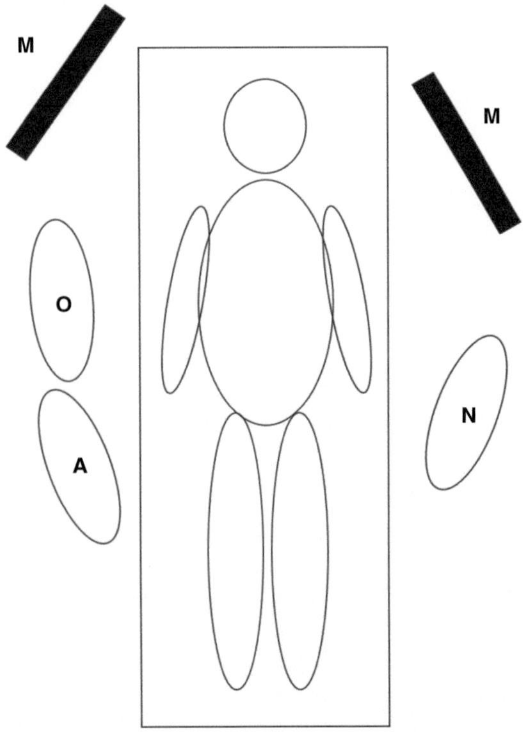

Fig. 15.1 Position of personnel and monitors. *O* operator, *A* assistant, *N* scrub nurse, *M* video monitor

The lateral decubitus position, as in conventional lung surgery, can also be used.

Instruments

Endoscopic instruments and 5-mm, 30° video thoracoscopy are used. Energy-based vessel sealing devices are more convenient than electrocautery for the dissection of mediastinal tissue and the division of small vessels. Endoscopic clips or staplers are necessary depending on the situation.

Ports Placement

The number of ports to use is a matter of preference. Single-port surgery, double-port surgery, and triple-port surgery can be performed safely and effectively [7, 9]. In multiport surgical procedures, only 3-mm or 5-mm ports are added compared with single-port surgery, and this does not increase clinically significant tissue damage or postoperative pain.

When performing triple-port surgery, the main procedure can be performed via three 5-mm ports, and the specimen can be removed through 1 of the ports after appropriate extension of the wound. In the bilateral approach, the preceding unilateral procedure is performed with three 5-mm ports on the ipsilateral side, and the specimen is removed via the contralateral side.

The first port is created in the fifth or sixth intercostal space in the mid-axillary line. After creating pneumothorax with single-lung ventilation and ambient air, a 5-mm trocar is introduced into the thoracic cavity. The thoracic cavity is inspected with a thoracoscope for potential adhesion, and CO_2 insufflation is started using a pressure limit of 8 mmHg. Under thoracoscopic guidance, trocars for additional ports are introduced into the third or fourth intercostal space in the anterior axillary line and into the fifth or sixth intercostal space along the midclavicular line. Any instrument can be inserted into any port according to the surgeon's preference and the situation. Usually, the scope is inserted through

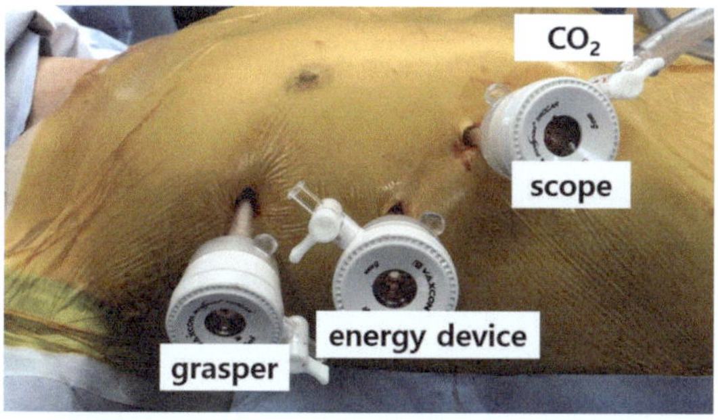

Fig. 15.2 Ports placement in triple-port surgery. Three ports were made in the fourth and sixth intercostal spaces with 5-mm trocars. Any instrument can be inserted via any port depending on the surgeon's preferences and the situation. The ipsilateral arm is dropped below the chest

lower ports (Fig. 15.2). In the left-side approach, the trocar in the superior port is inserted first to avoid cardiac injury. One incision is expanded at the end of the procedure according to the size of the specimen to be removed. In the case of single-port surgery, a 2- to 3-cm window is made in the fourth or fifth intercostal space in the anterior axillary line [9, 10]. An additional port is made in the third intercostal space in the anterior axillary line for double-port surgery.

Ports placement should be adjusted for each case, considering the extent of thymectomy and the patients' individual anatomical characteristics.

Thymectomy

Surgeons should have their own strategy for every step of thymectomy. The first step for thymectomy is identifying the anatomical landmarks and pathology of the thymus and making a plan for the case. The important landmarks of the anterior mediastinum in the lateral approach are the sternum ventrally, internal thoracic vein cranially, phrenic nerve dorsally, and diaphragm caudally. The mediastinal pleura is opened along with these structures. Dissection is usually carried out from the caudal to cranial direction. The main procedure starts with dissection of the substernal area to maximize the space. Care should be taken to protect the phrenic nerve while removing as much perithymic adipose tissue as possible, especially in myasthenia gravis patients. The innominate veins can be identified without difficulty by guidance of the internal thoracic veins (Fig. 15.3). The internal thoracic veins can be divided to facilitate exposure of the upper poles. The thymic veins should be dissected in full circumference, and the left brachiocephalic vein on the far side should be identified before division, especially when using energy-based vessel sealing devices, to avoid detrimental injuries to the left brachiocephalic vein. Only the upper part of the contralateral phrenic nerve can be identified from either side (Fig. 15.4). A complete dissection of contralateral diaphragmatic adipose tissue is impossible with the lateral

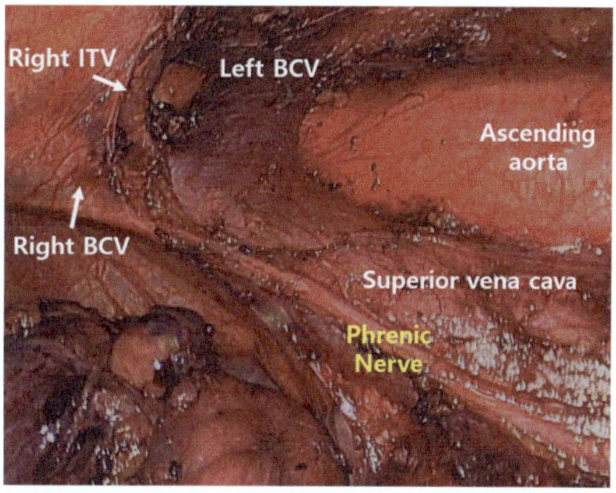

Fig. 15.3 Important anatomical structures in the right-side approach. *ITV* internal thoracic vein, *BCV* brachiocephalic vein

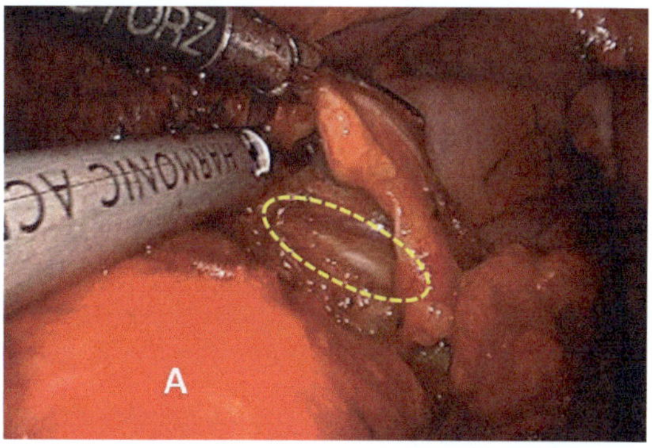

Fig. 15.4 The upper part of the left phrenic nerve (yellow-dotted area) can be identified during the right-side approach beyond the ascending aorta upon lifting the left mediastinal pleura. *A* ascending aorta

approach. Thus, a bilateral approach should be performed for extended thymectomy in myasthenia gravis. In the bilateral approach, it is preferential to start with the right-side approach with triple 5-mm ports. Dissection proceeds to the contralateral diaphragm as much as possible during the right-side operation, as dissection of the left diaphragmatic adipose tissue is relatively difficult due to the lower diaphragm position and left heart.

Whenever dense adhesion of the tumor to adjacent structures is encountered, en bloc resection should be attempted. Resection of the lung, pericardium, or phrenic nerves can be performed safely without difficulty. However, resection of other structures, such as great vessels and the chest wall, is not possible by VATS. A surgeon should be prepared for conversion to open surgery if the possibility of such involvement exists.

Lymph node dissection is recommended in thymic malignancies [5]. The perithymic, prevascular, and supradiaphragmatic nodes should be dissected routinely. The paratracheal (right-side approach) (Fig. 15.5) or paraaortic nodes (left-side approach) (Fig. 15.6) should be dissected in tumors invading other structures (≥T2) [11].

After completion of thymectomy, a small-bore drain is inserted through 1 port. If no bleeding is expected, placement of a drain can be omitted. Usually, 1 drain through the final side is sufficient in the bilateral approach.

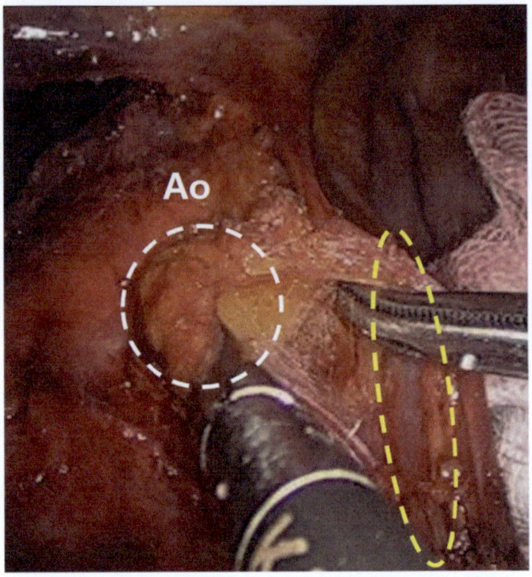

Fig. 15.6 The paraaortic node (white-dotted area) is pooled out beneath the left pericardiacophrenic neurovascular bundle (yellow-dotted area). *Ao* aortic arch

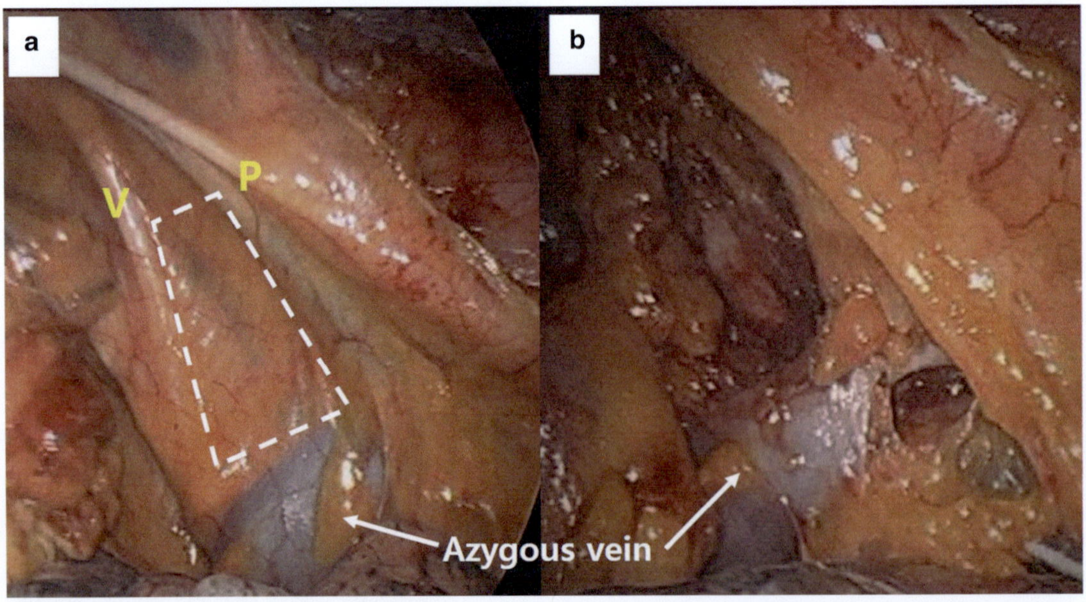

Fig. 15.5 (**a**) The right paratracheal area (white-dotted area) is accessible in the right-side approach. (**b**) Right paratracheal node dissection can be performed above and below the azygous vein. *V* vagus nerve, *P* phrenic nerve

Handling of Specimens

It is important to mark specific areas during resection on both the specimen side and in the patient. This allows a much more accurate interpretation of the specimen regarding the orientation and potential areas of concern. Marking in the patient facilitates communication with a radiation oncologist about specific areas of concern that may need to be addressed. Clear communication with pathologists about the orientation of the specimen is needed to accurately define resection margins and areas to target with adjuvant radiation [5].

15.3 Conclusion

Familiarity with the principles of the procedure, a precise preoperative evaluation, definitive surgical planning, and careful operation are required for successful VATS thymectomy.

Conflict of Interest No potential conflict of interest relevant to this article was reported.

References

1. Girard N, Ruffini E, Marx A, Faivre-Finn C, Peters S, ESMO Guidelines Committee. Thymic epithelial tumours: ESMO clinical practice guidelines for diagnosis, treatment and follow-up. Ann Oncol. 2015;26(Suppl 5):v40–55.
2. Narm KS, Lee CY, Do YW, et al. Limited thymectomy as a potential alternative treatment option for early-stage thymoma: a multi-institutional propensity-matched study. Lung Cancer. 2016;101:22–7.
3. Jaretzki A 3rd. Thymectomy for myasthenia gravis: analysis of controversies: patient management. Neurologist. 2003;9:77–92.
4. Toker A, Sonett J, Zielinski M, Rea F, Tomulescu V, Detterbeck FC. Standard terms, definitions, and policies for minimally invasive resection of thymoma. J Thorac Oncol. 2011;6(7 Suppl 3):S1739–42.
5. Detterbeck FC, Moran C, Huang J, et al. Which way is up? Policies and procedures for surgeons and pathologists regarding resection specimens of thymic malignancy. J Thorac Oncol. 2011;6(7 Suppl 3):S1730–8.
6. Liu Z, Yang R, Sun Y. Nonintubated uniportal thoracoscopic thymectomy with laryngeal mask. Thorac Cardiovasc Surg. 2020;68:450–6.
7. Bleetman D, West D, Teh E, Internullo E. Video-assisted thoracoscopic thymectomy. Ann Cardiothorac Surg. 2015;4:556–7.
8. Nakagiri T, Inoue M, Shintani Y, et al. Improved procedures and comparative results for video-assisted thoracoscopic extended thymectomy for myasthenia gravis. Surg Endosc. 2015;29:2859–65.
9. Ooi A, Sibayan M. Uniportal video assisted thoracoscopic surgery thymectomy (right approach). J Visc Surg. 2016;2:13.
10. Ooi A, Qiang F. Uniportal video assisted thoracoscopic surgery thymectomy (left approach). J Visc Surg. 2016;2:12.
11. Hwang Y, Park IK, Park S, Kim ER, Kang CH, Kim YT. Lymph node dissection in thymic malignancies: implication of the ITMIG lymph node map, TNM stage classification, and recommendations. J Thorac Oncol. 2016;11:108–14.

Video-Assisted Thoracic Surgery Thymectomy: Subxiphoid Approach

16

Sukki Cho

Abstract

Subxiphoid single-port video-assisted thoracic surgery (VATS) thymectomy is indicated for all anterior mediastinal masses and may be extended to lung cancer. The patient is placed in the lithotomy position, and the operator should be on the midline. Below the xiphoid process, a skin incision is made 4–5 cm horizontally at a single thumb's width down. Under 2-lung ventilation, CO_2 is insufflated, maintaining 10 mmHg. The fat tissue and thymic tissue are all resected from the sternum and pericardium between both phrenic nerves using an articulated grasper and an energy device. After retrieval of the mass with a wrap bag, a Jackson-Pratt drain is inserted instead of a chest tube. One of the advantages of this procedure is less postoperative pain than intercostal VATS. The subxiphoid approach can be used for bilateral pneumothorax, bilateral pulmonary metastasectomy, and simple lobectomy for both upper lobes and the right middle lobe.

S. Cho (✉)
Department of Thoracic and Cardiovascular Surgery, Seoul National University Bundang Hospital, Seoul National University College of Medicine, Seongnam, Gyeonggi-Do, Republic of Korea
e-mail: tubincho@snu.ac.kr

Keywords

Thymectomy · Subxiphoid · Video-assisted thoracic surgery · Single port

16.1 Introduction

Minimally invasive surgery for anterior mediastinal tumors includes the bilateral intercostal, cervical, and subxiphoid approaches. The intercostal approach was first performed by Landreneau et al. [1] in 1992, and is now the most popular approach. The cervical approach was initially performed by Cooper et al. [2] in 1988, but further use of this approach has not been reported in Korea. The subxiphoid approach was first performed by Kido et al. [3] in 1999 and was further advanced by Suda et al. [4]. In this paper, I would like to elaborate on single-port video-assisted thoracic surgery (VATS) thymectomy through the subxiphoid approach for anterior mediastinal tumors, with the goal of enabling beginners to perform this procedure safely.

16.2 Indications

This method is indicated for almost all anterior mediastinal masses, except masses with vascular invasion (especially invasive thymomas). Funnel chest, cardiomegaly, and a large tumor (>5 cm)

K. Kim et al. (eds.), *Techniques in Minimally Invasive Thoracic Surgery*,
https://doi.org/10.1007/978-981-19-2472-9_16

are relative contraindications. In addition to anterior mediastinal masses, this approach is also highly suitable for lymph node metastasis to the internal mammary chain or cardiophrenic angle. Some surgeons have used this technique for lung cancer surgery, but in my opinion, doing so is premature because of the great difficulty of performing both lower lobectomy and subcarinal lymph node dissection, similar to the conventional VATS procedure.

16.3 Anatomy of the Subxiphoid Area

The anterior mediastinum is located between the body of the sternum in the front and the anterior pericardium posteriorly (Fig. 16.1). It contains loose connective tissue, mediastinal fat, and the body of the thymus.

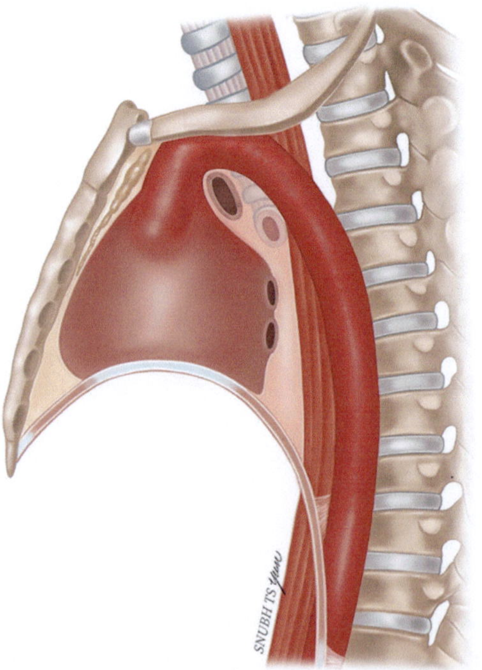

Fig. 16.1 Mediastinum. The anterior mediastinum is located between the body of the sternum in the front and the anterior pericardium posteriorly

16.4 Procedure

Anesthesia

In principle, a single-lumen endotracheal tube can be used because 1-lung ventilation is not necessary. However, it is convenient to use a double-lumen endotracheal tube if the tumor is large or lung invasion is suspected. Intensive arterial monitoring is required because of the possibility of CO_2 retention with CO_2 insufflation and cardiac compromise during surgery or when the tumor is removed. Because the operation time is not long, it is not necessary to insert a Foley catheter or to catheterize the femoral, jugular, or subclavian vein in the absence of vascular invasion.

Position

The lithotomy position is preferable because the operator should be on the midline (Fig. 16.2). Both arms should be at attention because sternotomy may be required in some situations. The drape can expose the upper abdomen, sternal notch, and mid-axillary line on both sides.

Surgical Instruments

1. Wound retractor.
2. Multiport (Lapsingle version).
3. 30° thoracoscope (5 mm or 10 mm).
4. Grasper (5 mm), as long as possible (>30 cm): an articulating grasper is the best, such as the artisential grasper.
5. Energy device: Ligasure, a Harmonic scalpel, or Thunderbeat are options, but if possible, the Maryland tip shape is preferable and it should be as long as possible (>35 cm).
6. Vinyl bag, medium or large size.

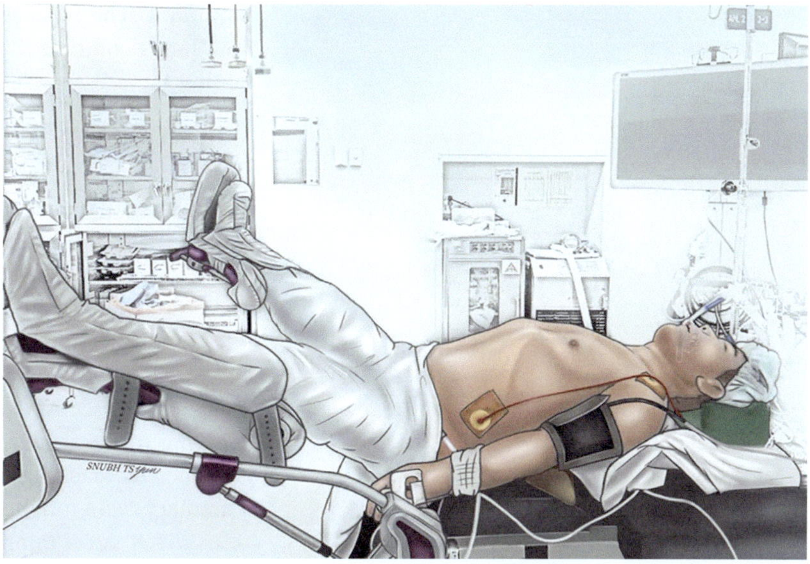

Fig. 16.2 Patient position. The lithotomy position is preferable, and the operator stands between the patient's legs

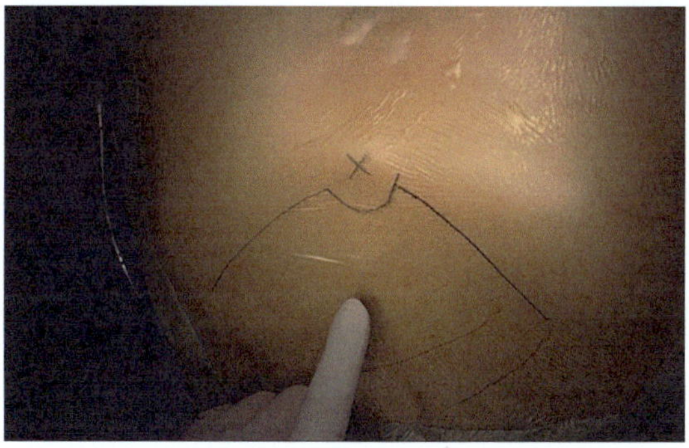

Fig. 16.3 Skin incision. A 5-cm horizontal incision is made below the xiphoid process

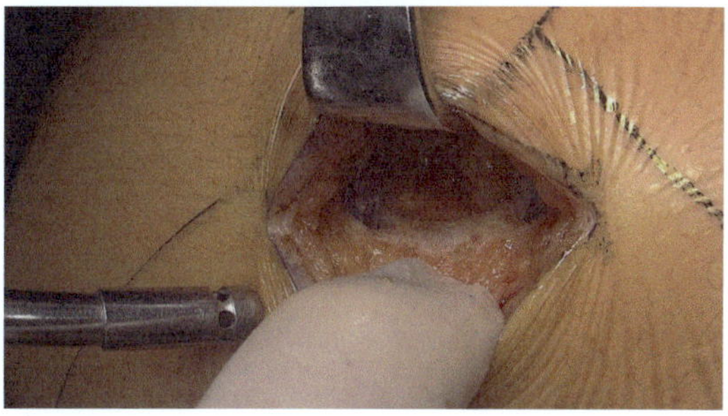

Fig. 16.4 Before port placement. The rectus muscle is transected about 1 cm horizontally and further dissection is performed 360° under the xiphoid process

Incision and Port Placement

Incision (Fig. 16.3)

A skin incision is made 4–5 cm horizontally at a single thumb's width down from the xiphoid process. At first, it is better to be sure to make a long enough incision, and the incision size can then be gradually reduced with practice. There are two methods of skin incision: vertical and horizontal. The advantages of a vertical incision are that it is possible not to transect the rectus muscle, and if sternotomy is also performed, the skin incision is connected. The advantage of a horizontal incision is that it spreads slightly better on the lateral side, thus reducing collisions between instruments within a single port. Therefore, the choice between a vertical and horizontal incision should be made according to the situation.

Port Placement

After finding the xiphoid process, the rectus muscle is transected about 1 cm to both sides and further dissection is performed 360° under the xiphoid process (Fig. 16.4). Using the index finger as in sternotomy, sufficient additional dissection is performed under the sternum. Adding a wound protector, the subxiphoid area is further dissected using a monopolar Bovie under thoracoscopic guidance. The Lapsingle is added and CO_2 insufflation is started, maintaining 10 mmHg (Fig. 16.5). The position of the multiport and the location of the port for instruments are very

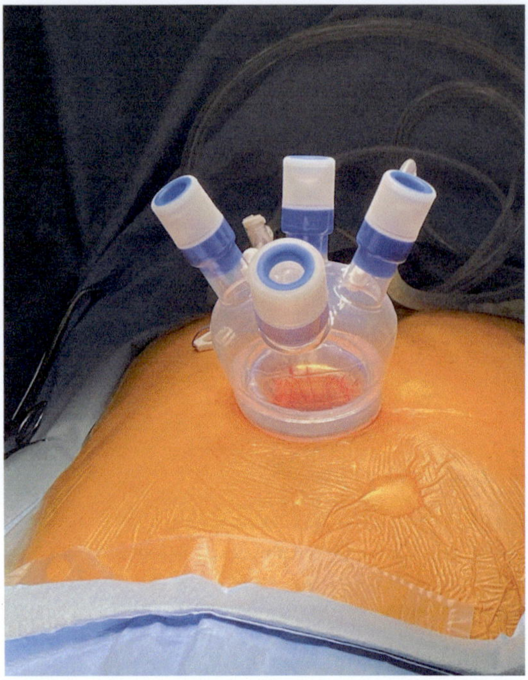

Fig. 16.5 After port placement. The multiport is added and CO_2 insufflation is started, maintaining 10 mmHg

important. The bilateral pleurae are opened and both lungs continue to be ventilated while maintaining the pressure of CO_2 at around 10 mmHg (Fig. 16.6).

Thymectomy

When sufficient space is available for the subxiphoid approach, the next step is to drop the thymic tissue from the sternum. The boundary between the two sides is formed by the mammary vein, and dissection proceeds upward, closely adhering to the sternum. The mediastinal pleura is opened by reaching as far as possible where the mammary vein on both sides inserts into the veins. After confirming that there is no bleeding, the thymic and pericardial fat is again dissected, as well as pleural fat from the inlet of the incision. If myasthenia gravis (MG) is present, more complete dissection will be necessary. During dissection, it is necessary to check the course of both phrenic nerves (Fig. 16.7). In particular, if

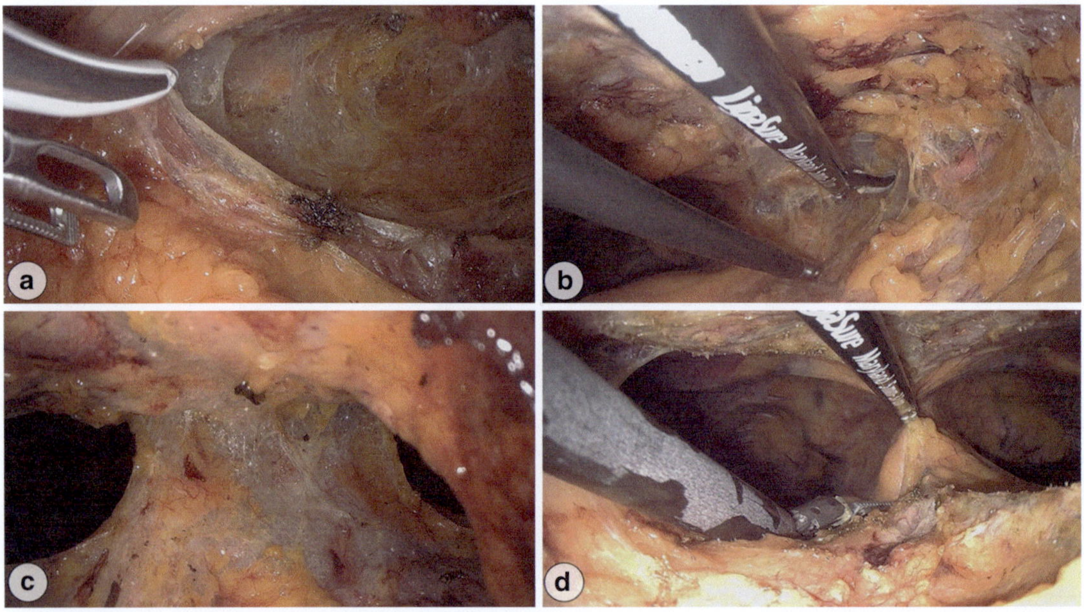

Fig. 16.6 Open pleura. (**a**) Dissection of the substernal tissue using an energy device, (**b**) opening of the right pleura, (**c**) opening of the left pleura, (**d**) dissection of the substernal thymic tissue

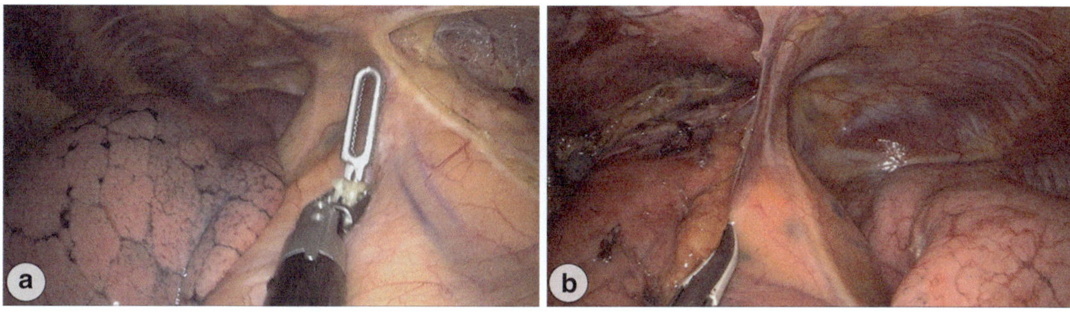

Fig. 16.7 Phrenic nerve. (**a**) Right phrenic nerve, (**b**) left phrenic nerve

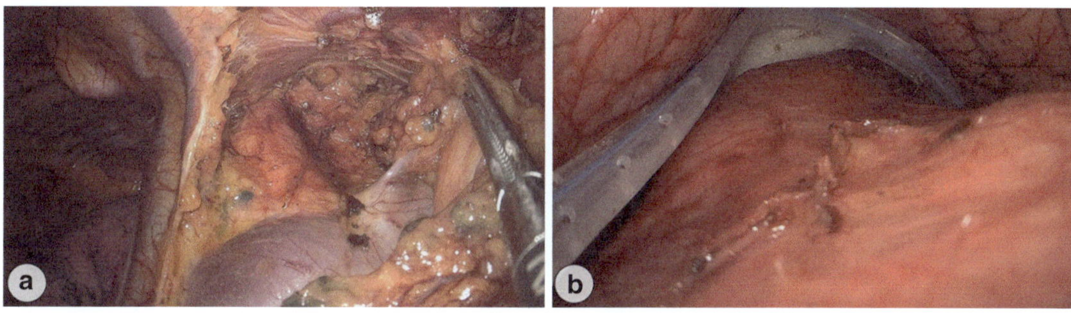

Fig. 16.8 Thymectomy. (**a**) Both upper poles are removed, (**b**) a Jackson-Pratt drain is positioned after retrieval of the mass

there is a suspicion that the thymic tumor invades the surrounding organs, they should be resected together to the greatest extent possible. Since it is quite possible for both lungs to have adhesions or invasions, an endostapler is used to resect them en bloc instead of being forced to dissect them from the mass. When encountering the innominate vein, the thymic tissue is lifted and one proceeds upward while dissecting the front of the vein. There is no branch in this area, so there is no major problem with dissecting the vessel. Next, the left upper pole is dissected. The reason for this is that if the operator is right-handed, it seems safer empirically. Furthermore, since the left pole is larger than the right, one can think of the point of removing the left pole as the farthest place during surgery. Small branches can be clipped, but this step may vary depending on the energy device used. CO_2 insufflation is usually used, so it may seem that there are no areas of small bleeding, but when CO_2 is cut off at the end of surgery, bleeding may occur; therefore, I recommend using a clip if possible. The left pole is removed from the top of the innominate vein, one proceeds to the right, the tissue is dissected in front of the trachea, and the right pole is removed from the front of the left innominate artery.

After total thymectomy, a wrap bag is inserted through one of the multiports, and the thymus, including the mass and adjacent fat tissue, is retrieved from the chest. It is important to note that if the tumor is large and hard, it will press upon the heart as it is removed through a narrow space; therefore, the patient's blood pressure and heart rhythm should be carefully observed.

When observing the surgical field after removing the tumor, there is no temporary CO_2 in the thoracic cavity, so if there is a blood vessel for which proper hemostasis was not achieved, bleeding is visible. In the absence of bleeding, depending on the intraoperative findings of thymic disease, it is recommended to check for pleural metastasis under 1-lung ventilation. There is no need to insert a chest tube; at this point, I insert a Jackson-Pratt (J-P) drain and close the surgical field layer by layer (Fig. 16.8).

Postoperative Management

Immediately after the operation, a chest posteroanterior radiograph should be checked in the operating room to determine whether there is pneumothorax. If pneumothorax is present, temporary suction can be applied to the J-P drain until the air leak is stopped. On postoperative day 1, the amount and color of the drainage are checked. If there is no evidence of chyle and the amount is less than 200 mL, the J-P drain is removed. Special medications, including painkillers, are not necessary unless the patient has MG.

16.5 Advantages

One of the advantages of this approach is that it can reduce the frequency of bleeding caused by damage to the innominate vein, and the probability of successful hemostasis is very high without an open procedure because of the good visibility. In addition, it is very easy to perform median sternotomy without changing the patient's position when it is difficult to proceed with the subxiphoid approach.

In the 1-sided VATS approach, if there are pleural adhesions, almost all adhesions must be released, and the air leakage is often severe due to lung damage caused by adhesiolysis. However, the subxiphoid approach does not cause lung damage because only a small amount of adhesiolysis gives enough vision of the area to be operated on; therefore, chest tube insertion is not required.

Postoperative pain is also an inevitable complication even after 1-sided VATS. However, the subxiphoid approach causes significantly less postoperative pain than 1-sided VATS, because the intercostal nerve is not damaged by the surgical instruments during surgery, and the intercostal or other thoracic muscles are not incised.

16.6 Disadvantages

A special instrument is required to operate in a narrow space. Most of the instruments used in VATS procedures are straight, so surgery is very difficult for patients with an exceptionally depressed sternum. Thus, it can be very useful to have instruments with multiple types of articulations. Although energy devices have a straight body, there is no particular inconvenience because the tip is curved.

Suction cannot be used freely because CO_2 insufflation is required. There is a risk of cardiac and pulmonary compromise depending on the pressure and flow of CO_2.

16.7 Conclusion

In the near future, the subxiphoid approach can be applied to bilateral pneumothorax, bilateral pulmonary metastasectomy (especially for metastases on both upper lobes), and simple lobectomy for both upper lobes and the right middle lobe.

Conflict of Interest No potential conflict of interest relevant to this article was reported.

References

1. Landreneau RJ, Dowling RD, Castillo WM, Ferson PF. Thoracoscopic resection of an anterior mediastinal tumor. Ann Thorac Surg. 1992;54:142–4.
2. Cooper JD, Al-Jilaihawa AN, Pearson FG, Humphrey JG, Humphrey HE. An improved technique to facilitate transcervical thymectomy for myasthenia gravis. Ann Thorac Surg. 1988;45:242–7.
3. Kido T, Hazama K, Inoue Y, Tanaka Y, Takao T. Resection of anterior mediastinal masses through an infrasternal approach. Ann Thorac Surg. 1999;67:263–5.
4. Suda T, Sugimura H, Tochii D, Kihara M, Hattori Y. Single-port thymectomy through an infrasternal approach. Ann Thorac Surg. 2012;93:334–6.

Robot-Assisted Thoracic Surgery Thymectomy

17

Samina Park

Abstract

Robotic thymectomy has been adopted recently and has been shown to be safe and feasible in treating thymic tumors and myasthenia gravis. The surgical indications of robotic technology are expanding, with advantages including an excellent surgical view and sophisticated manipulation. Herein, we describe technical aspects, considerations, and outcomes of robotic thymectomy.

Keywords

Robotic surgery · Thymectomy · Minimally invasive surgery · Thymic neoplasms Myasthenia gravis

17.1 Introduction

The minimally invasive approach has emerged as an alternative to median sternotomy for thymectomy. Minimally invasive thymectomy has been widely performed using thoracoscopy [1–4]. Since the first robotic thymectomy was reported in 2003 by Ashton et al. [5], it has been widely accepted as an effective surgical option for thymic epithelial tumors (TET) and myasthenia gravis (MG) [6–9]. From the standpoint of surgical outcomes, robotic thymectomy has shown excellent safety and perioperative results, with comparable outcomes to open sternotomy in terms of oncologic survival and neurologic improvement [1, 2, 9–11]. Robotic thymectomy is commonly performed via the lateral or subxiphoid approach [12–15]. Technical advances in robotic surgery have expanded the indications for robotic thymectomy. Furthermore, single-port and single-site platforms are also applied for treating anterior mediastinal masses [16–18]. In this article, technical details, considerations, and outcomes of robotic thymectomy are described.

S. Park (✉)
Department of Thoracic and Cardiovascular Surgery, Seoul National University Hospital, Seoul National University College of Medicine, Seoul, Republic of Korea
e-mail: sam841203@snu.ac.kr

17.2 Surgical Anatomy

The thymus is a lymphoid organ located in the anterior part of the superior mediastinum, extending into the anterior mediastinum. It is composed of two lobes covered with loose connective tissue. The thymus lies behind the sternum and strap muscles, and anterior to the pericardium, the innominate vein, superior vena cava, ascending aorta, aortic arch, and arch vessels. It is connected to the lower poles of the thyroid gland by the thyrothymic ligament. Laterally, the phrenic nerves and mediastinal pleura run along the thymus bilaterally. The thymic arteries mainly comprise (1) the lateral thymic artery from the internal

K. Kim et al. (eds.), *Techniques in Minimally Invasive Thoracic Surgery*,
https://doi.org/10.1007/978-981-19-2472-9_17

mammary artery and the pericardiacophrenic artery, (2) the superior thymic artery from the inferior thyroid artery, and (3) the posterior thymic artery from the aorta or innominate artery. The thymic veins comprise (1) the posterior thymic vein to the innominate vein, and (2) small tributaries to the inferior thyroid vein, internal mammary vein, and superior vena cava. The lymphatic vessels drain to the parasternal, brachiocephalic, and tracheobronchial lymph nodes.

17.3 Indications

Total thymectomy is primarily indicated for TET and MG [19, 20]. Based on institutional experience, en bloc resection of the invaded organs, including the pericardium, lung, phrenic nerve, and innominate vein, is safely performed by robotic thymectomy. However, advanced thymic tumors invading the chest wall or great vessels and large tumors (over 8 cm) are considered contraindications of robotic thymectomy [15, 21].

17.4 Procedure

Robotic Thymectomy Via the Subxiphoid Approach

Using robotic technology in addition to the subxiphoid approach may maximize the advantages of the subxiphoid approach by enabling meticulous dissection and safe manipulation around the upper mediastinum, even in advanced tumors. Since robotic thymectomy via the subxiphoid approach (RTX) was reported by Suda et al. [22], several advantages of the subxiphoid approach in thymectomy have been suggested, including (1) an excellent view of the bilateral upper poles of the thymus and bilateral phrenic nerves, (2) minimal pain from not spreading the intercostal space, and (3) excellent cosmesis [4, 14, 23, 24]. Herein, the details of RTX are described.

Preparation

A double-lumen endotracheal tube is routinely used during thymectomy, but single-lung ventilation is limited to selective application in cases involving concomitant lung resection and/or identification of the dislocated phrenic nerve due to a large tumor. Central catheterization is not used. The patient is positioned supine with a 10-cm depth of the pad under the back and both arms abducted to prevent interference with the movement of the robotic arms (Fig. 17.1). The table is not tilted and the patient is not placed in the reverse Trendelenburg position. No additional instrument for sternal elevation is used. Figure 17.2 shows a typical port placement for 3-arm RTX. A 3- to 4-cm vertical incision is made at the lower half of the xiphoid process. After dividing the linea alba, the xiphoid process is partially resected to widen the subxiphoid space and reduce collisions between the camera arm and the sternum. The bilateral mediastinal pleura is opened using electrocautery under thoracoscopic guidance while an assistant holds the sternum upward to ensure sufficient space between the sternum and pericardium (Fig. 17.2). Then, a 4-channel glove port inserted through the subxiphoid window allows CO_2 insufflation, which makes a wide substernal space and collapses the lungs through the pleural opening. Two additional robotic ports are safely inserted at the bilateral fifth intercostal space along the midpoint between the midclavicular line and the anterior axillary line (Fig. 17.3). Most thymectomies can be completed using the 3-arm technique (Maryland bipolar forceps for the first robotic

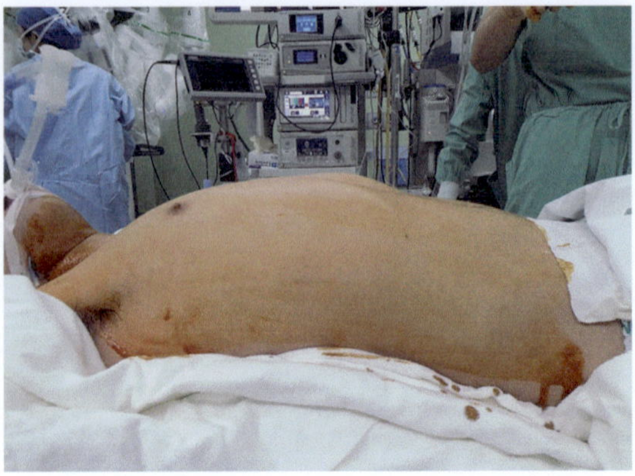

Fig. 17.1 The patient is positioned supine with a 10-cm depth of the pad under the back and both arms abducted

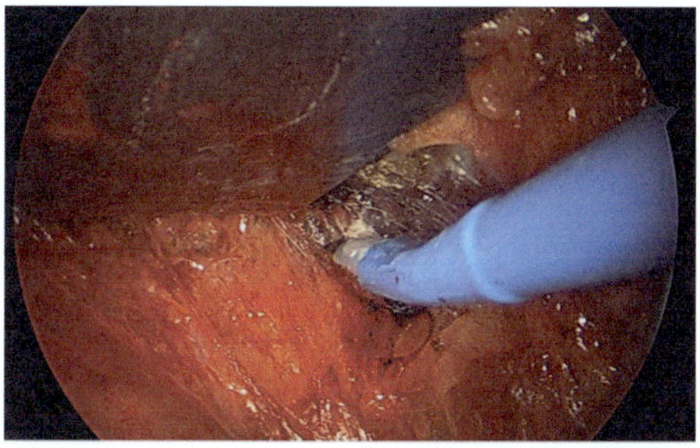

Fig. 17.2 The bilateral mediastinal pleura is opened using electrocautery under thoracoscopic guidance

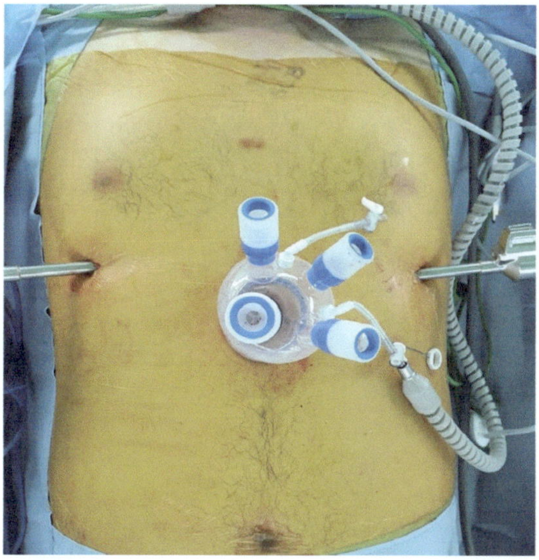

Fig. 17.3 Typical port placement for 3-arm robotic thymectomy via the subxiphoid approach

arm, 30° camera for the second arm, and Harmonic ACE curved shears or Monopolar curved scissors [Hot Shears] for the third arm); however, advanced cases require an additional holding arm (Force bipolar for the fourth arm), which is placed in the third or fourth intercostal space at the anterior axillary line. After docking the robot, the patient cart is placed above the patient's head. The da Vinci Si System can be used for the subxiphoid approach in most cases, but it cannot be utilized effectively in some advanced cases. Moreover, the 12-mm camera of the Si System induces frequent collisions between the sternum and the camera and reduces the flexibility to approach the patient's bed from multiple directions. Therefore, to benefit from the advantages of the subxiphoid approach, the da Vinci Xi System is more suitable than the Si System.

Retrosternal Dissection and Pleural Cavity Exploration

The thymus is separated with Harmonic ACE curved shears from the sternum via 30° upward vision. The strap muscles and bilateral internal mammary vessels are useful anatomical boundaries for total thymectomy. Then, the angle of the camera turns to 30° down and the bilateral pleural cavity should be explored to identify unexpected pleural seeding nodules, tumor invasion to adjacent organs, and the location of the bilateral phrenic nerves.

Dissection of the Bilateral Upper Poles and Innominate Vein

Upper pole dissection is relatively difficult in the lateral approach. However, in the subxiphoid approach, the trachea, the innominate artery, and the sternal notch are easily accessible without collision of instruments or limited vision. Complete dissection of the bilateral upper poles from the thyroid gland is possible in most cases (Fig. 17.4). The thymic vasculature is relatively inconsistent. However, most thymic vessels are small enough to be divided with a robotic energy device. Bipolar electrocautery or ligation clips can also be applied according to the surgeon's

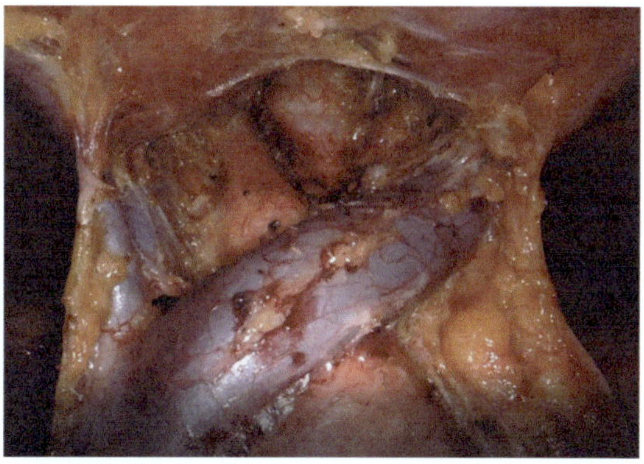

Fig. 17.4 After dissecting the bilateral upper poles and innominate vein, the upper mediastinum is clearly exposed

preference. In addition, the Harmonic ACE curved shears for the third arm is not an angulated device; therefore, dissection from the left lobe to the right lobe is helpful for safely dividing venous tributaries draining to the innominate vein.

Dissection of Bilateral Lower Poles

Separation of the lower poles of the thymus from the pericardium can be easily performed with a robotic energy device. For small tumors without invasion of the adjacent organs, the entire procedure is conducted with a robotic energy device. In cases of tumors abutting or invading the phrenic nerves or the pericardium, robotic monopolar curved scissors are suitable for a precise dissection. In addition, the robotic camera can be inserted laterally in the contralateral direction through the subxiphoid window to improve the exposure of the diaphragmatic fat.

Specimen Retrieval

While CO_2 gas is insufflated, the endo bag through one channel of a glove port is placed in the pleural cavity under the guidance of the robotic camera inserted in the port for the first robotic arm. The resected thymus is brought into the endo bag using the third robotic arm to avoid injuring the tumor or adjacent organs. Then, the specimen is retrieved via the subxiphoid window. Additional extension of the wound is rarely required because the substernal space is quite flexible.

Advantages of RTX

RTX enables extensive resection and meticulous dissection in stage II–III TET and tumors located in the upper mediastinum. Therefore, the following potential advantages of RTX over other minimally invasive approaches are suggested.

Easy to Learn

The surgical view is similar to traditional sternotomy. In addition, the instruments used during the procedure are simple enough to be familiar and the assistant's help is rarely required. Furthermore, if open sternotomy is required, the subxiphoid window can immediately be extended to median sternotomy. Therefore, novice surgeons who would like to start performing robotic thoracic surgery are recommended to start with RTX for small tumors as their first robotic procedure.

Feasible for Advanced or Large Tumors

The excellent exposure of the superior mediastinum from the subxiphoid approach, in addition to the advantages of the robotic technique, allows surgeons to perform a fine dissection for complete resection and complex procedures such as reconstruction of the pericardium, vessels, and nerves, which were previously considered to require open sternotomy [25, 26]. (1) Pericardium: Pericardial resection and reconstruction can easily be completed with robotic instruments. Pericardial defects are reconstructed with a Gore-Tex membrane using a robotic needle driver. The preferred suture materials are silk and polypropylene. (2) Lung: En bloc wedge resection of the invaded lung is carried with robotic staplers (Fig. 17.5). If concomitant lobectomy during RTX is needed for a tumor invading the pulmonary hilum, the modified subxiphoid approach can be applied [27]. (3) Innominate vein: The innominate vein can be transected or partially resected with robotic staplers (Fig. 17.6). If the innominate vein should be reconstructed, vascular clamps are useful to control the proximal and

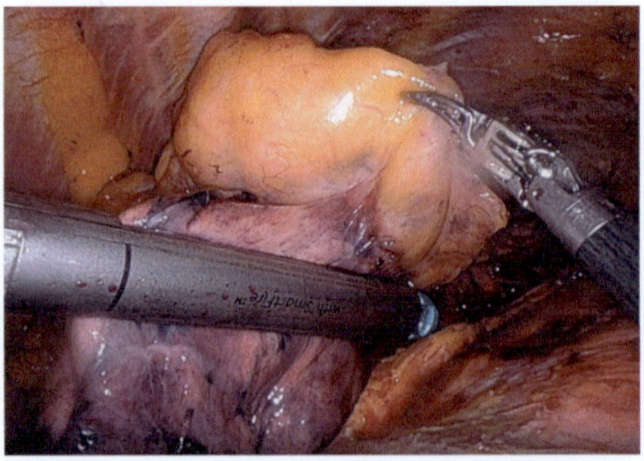

Fig. 17.5 A robotic stapler is used for en bloc wedge resection of the right upper lobe during robotic thymectomy

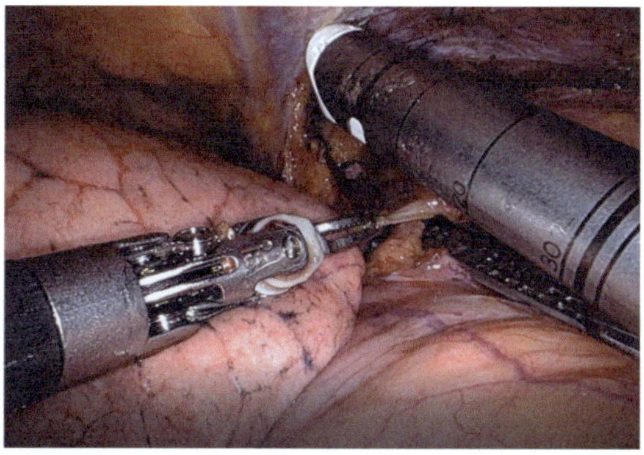

Fig. 17.6 The proximal innominate vein is divided with a robotic stapler

distal part of the vessel during the reconstruction using a vascular prosthesis [25]. (4) Phrenic nerve: Firefly vision is useful to find pericardiacophrenic vessels if the phrenic nerve is not clearly defined in obese patients or tumors overriding the nerve [28]. Neurorrhaphy is also feasible using robotic technology for a partially resected phrenic nerve.

Easy to Modify

Some modifications can be made by changing the location of the ports and the direction of the approach. According to the location or size of tumors, inserting the robotic camera into the ipsilateral thoracic cavity through the fifth intercostal space is an alternative method (modified subxiphoid approach) [27]. Furthermore, the camera inserted through the intercostal port provides an excellent surgical view around the tumor and the pulmonary hilum. It also can be modified to uniportal surgery using a single-site platform for limited cases [17].

Feasible for Lymph Node Dissection

Anterior (perithymic) lymph nodes (N1) can be removed during total thymectomy. However, deep regional lymph nodes (N2) cannot be dissected using conventional minimally invasive approaches due to the limited surgical view. However, the right and left paratracheal areas can be safely accessed by RTX. The subcarinal area can be approached through the modified subxiphoid approach.

Preserves the Intercostal Space and Bundles

An important aspect of the subxiphoid approach is its ability to spare the intercostal muscles and bundles, which is associated with reducing intercostal neuralgia. Unlike the lateral approach, large tumors can be retrieved via a subxiphoid window without additional extension of the wound in most cases.

Robotic Thymectomy Via the Lateral Approach

Robotic thymectomy via the lateral approach has been more commonly performed than RTX. The lateral approach is performed via the right side, left side, or bilaterally, according to the extent and location of the mass or the surgeon's preference. However, the bilateral approach is generally preferred for patients with MG. The patient is placed in the supine position with elevation of the side to be approached. The adduction and lower positioning of the ipsilateral arm enable the robotic arm and trocar near the axilla to move more freely without injuring the patient by pressing. The 3-arm technique is commonly used. The camera port is inserted at the fourth or fifth intercostal space along the mid-axillary line. Then, CO_2 gas is insufflated under single-lung ventilation. CO_2 insufflation is mandatory during the entire procedure and provides a wide substernal space to manipulate the dissected thymus under clear vision. The pressure is initially 5 mmHg and is increased to 12 mmHg gradually under stable vital signs, if required. The instruments used are Maryland bipolar forceps for the first robotic arm at the fourth or fifth intercostal space along the mid-axillary line, and Harmonic ACE curved shears or monopolar curved scissors for the third arm at the fifth or sixth intercostal space along the anterior axillary line. An assistant for the suction device can be additionally used between the camera port and third arm port, if necessary. After docking of the robotic arms, thymectomy is performed in the same manner through conventional thoracoscopic thymectomy via the lateral approach. Therefore, skillful thoracoscopic surgeons may be familiar with the adoption of robotic techniques in thymectomy via the lateral approach.

17.5 Postoperative Management

A single Jackson–Pratt drain is placed across the substernal area and is removed on the operative day. Patients are usually discharged on the day after surgery. When concomitant lung resection is performed, a chest tube is inserted. Patients who are expected to have respiratory difficulty due to MG or phrenic nerve resection should only be managed in the intensive care unit.

17.6 Outcomes of Robotic Thymectomy

The safety and feasibility of robotic thymectomy for TET have been reported, with a complication rate less than 5% [14, 15, 21, 22, 24]. In addition, oncologic outcomes were satisfactory (5-year disease-specific survival of 100% in thymoma and 95% in thymic carcinoma) [21]. Neurological benefits and decreased use of steroids in MG were observed after robotic thymectomy (complete remission rates of 39% in robotic thymectomy and 20% in nonrobotic thymectomy) [29, 30]. No studies have yet compared the subxiphoid and lateral approaches in robotic thymectomy. However, it is reasonable to predict that RTX would be more suitable for advanced and highly located tumors due to the innate characteristics of RTX. Two meta-analyses of thoracoscopic thymectomy revealed that the subxiphoid approach was associated with less blood loss, a lower pain score, and a shorter hospital stay compared to the lateral approach [31, 32]. Furthermore, there were no differences in conversion to open sternotomy and oncologic outcomes between the two approaches [31]. Randomized studies comparing open sternotomy, the thoracoscopic approach, and the robotic approach would seem to have difficulty in enrolling patients in practice because the indications for each approach are quite different. Obviously, considering the maximal utilization of robotic techniques in thymectomy, more extensive thymectomy would be available than with thoracoscopic thymectomy.

17.7 Conclusion

Median sternotomy was the gold standard in thymectomy for decades. However, minimally invasive thymectomy has gained popularity because it has demonstrated comparable outcomes to those of open sternotomy. More recently, the robotic approach has become widely adopted in thymectomy. In addition, the subxiphoid approach, which provides an excellent surgical view for highly located tumors and the bilateral phrenic nerves, has been introduced. Thymectomy should be conducted following oncologic principles, regardless of the surgical technique. Furthermore, cosmetic benefits never take precedence over safe and complete surgery. Therefore, surgeons should be familiar with the features of various surgical techniques and utilize the advantages of each approach during thymectomy. The superiority of robotic thymectomy over other minimally invasive approaches or the lateral approach should be investigated in the future.

Conflict of Interest No potential conflict of interest relevant to this article was reported.

References

1. Jurado J, Javidfar J, Newmark A, et al. Minimally invasive thymectomy and open thymectomy: outcome analysis of 263 patients. Ann Thorac Surg. 2012;94:974–81.
2. Cheng YJ, Kao EL, Chou SH. Videothoracoscopic resection of stage II thymoma: prospective comparison of the results between thoracoscopy and open methods. Chest. 2005;128:3010–2.
3. Kido T, Hazama K, Inoue Y, Tanaka Y, Takao T. Resection of anterior mediastinal masses through an infrasternal approach. Ann Thorac Surg. 1999;67:263–5.
4. Suda T, Sugimura H, Tochii D, Kihara M, Hattori Y. Single-port thymectomy through an infrasternal approach. Ann Thorac Surg. 2012;93:334–6.

5. Ashton RC Jr, McGinnis KM, Connery CP, Swistel DG, Ewing DR, DeRose JJ Jr. Totally endoscopic robotic thymectomy for myasthenia gravis. Ann Thorac Surg. 2003;75:569–71.
6. Marulli G, Rea F, Melfi F, et al. Robot-aided thoracoscopic thymectomy for early-stage thymoma: a multicenter European study. J Thorac Cardiovasc Surg. 2012;144:1125–30.
7. Marulli G, Schiavon M, Perissinotto E, et al. Surgical and neurologic outcomes after robotic thymectomy in 100 consecutive patients with myasthenia gravis. J Thorac Cardiovasc Surg. 2013;145:730–5.
8. Ismail M, Swierzy M, Ruckert JC. State of the art of robotic thymectomy. World J Surg. 2013;37:2740–6.
9. Ye B, Li W, Ge XX, et al. Surgical treatment of early-stage thymomas: robot-assisted thoracoscopic surgery versus transsternal thymectomy. Surg Endosc. 2014;28:122–6.
10. Kang CH, Hwang Y, Lee HJ, Park IK, Kim YT. Robotic thymectomy in anterior mediastinal mass: propensity score matching study with transsternal thymectomy. Ann Thorac Surg. 2016;102:895–901.
11. Meyer DM, Herbert MA, Sobhani NC, et al. Comparative clinical outcomes of thymectomy for myasthenia gravis performed by extended transsternal and minimally invasive approaches. Ann Thorac Surg. 2009;87:385–90.
12. Chen K, Zhang X, Jin R, et al. Robot-assisted thoracoscopic surgery for mediastinal masses: a single-institution experience. J Thorac Dis. 2020;12:105–13.
13. Suda T, Kaneda S, Hachimaru A, et al. Thymectomy via a subxiphoid approach: single-port and robot-assisted. J Thorac Dis. 2016;8(Suppl 3):S265–71.
14. Zhang H, Chen L, Zheng Y, et al. Robot-assisted thymectomy via subxiphoid approach: technical details and early outcomes. J Thorac Dis. 2018;10:1677–82.
15. Kang CH, Na KJ, Song JW, et al. The robotic thymectomy via the subxiphoid approach: technique and early outcomes. Eur J Cardiothorac Surg. 2020;58(Suppl_1):i39–43.
16. Ishikawa N, Oda M, Kawachi K, Watanabe G. Robot-assisted single-port surgery for mediastinal tumors. Surg Today. 2019;49:96–8.
17. Park SY, Han KN, Hong JI, Kim HK, Kim DJ, Choi YH. Subxiphoid approach for robotic single-site-assisted thymectomy. Eur J Cardiothorac Surg. 2020;58(Suppl_1):i34–8.
18. Park SY, Kim HK, Jang DS, Han KN, Kim DJ. Initial experiences with robotic single-site thoracic surgery for mediastinal masses. Ann Thorac Surg. 2019;107:242–7.
19. Wolfe GI, Kaminski HJ, Aban IB, et al. Randomized trial of thymectomy in myasthenia gravis. N Engl J Med. 2016;375:511–22.
20. Ettinger DS, Riely GJ, Akerley W, et al. Thymomas and thymic carcinomas: clinical practice guidelines in oncology. J Natl Compr Canc Netw. 2013;11:562–76.
21. Kang CH, Na KJ, Park S, Park IK, Kim YT. Long-term outcomes of robotic thymectomy in patients with thymic epithelial tumors. Ann Thorac Surg. 2020;112(2):430–5. https://doi.org/10.1016/j.athoracsur.2020.09.018.
22. Suda T, Tochii D, Tochii S, Takagi Y. Trans-subxiphoid robotic thymectomy. Interact Cardiovasc Thorac Surg. 2015;20:669–71.
23. Chiu CH, Chao YK, Liu YH. Subxiphoid approach for video-assisted thoracoscopic surgery: an update. J Thorac Dis. 2018;10(Suppl 14):S1662–5.
24. Hashimoto K, Sakamaki H. The technical aspects of a midline robotic thymectomy. JTCVS Tech. 2020;4:368–70.
25. Suda T, Nagano H, Kawai H, Hoshikawa Y. Subxiphoid robot-assisted thymectomy with vascular prosthetic replacement. Semin Thorac Cardiovasc Surg. 2020;32:1133–4.
26. Na KJ, Kang CH. Neurorrhaphy of the phrenic nerve injury during robotic thymectomy. ASVIDE; 2020. https://www.asvide.com/article/view/33088. Accessed 30 May 2021.
27. Na KJ, Kang CH. Robotic thymectomy for advanced thymic epithelial tumor: indications and technical aspects. J Thorac Dis. 2020;12:63–9.
28. Wagner OJ, Louie BE, Vallieres E, Aye RW, Farivar AS. Near-infrared fluorescence imaging can help identify the contralateral phrenic nerve during robotic thymectomy. Ann Thorac Surg. 2012;94:622–5.
29. Keijzers M, de Baets M, Hochstenbag M, et al. Robotic thymectomy in patients with myasthenia gravis: neurological and surgical outcomes. Eur J Cardiothorac Surg. 2015;48:40–5.
30. Ruckert JC, Swierzy M, Ismail M. Comparison of robotic and nonrobotic thoracoscopic thymectomy: a cohort study. J Thorac Cardiovasc Surg. 2011;141:673–7.
31. Li J, Qi G, Liu Y, Zheng X, Zhang X. Meta-analysis of subxiphoid approach versus lateral approach for thoracoscopic thymectomy. J Cardiothorac Surg. 2020;15:89.
32. Li M, Xu L, Li L, Dai Q, Xu D. The early perioperative outcomes of subxiphoid approach versus lateral intercostal approach thoracoscopic thymectomy for thymic tumors: a meta-analysis. J Laparoendosc Adv Surg Tech A. 2021;32(3):256–64. https://doi.org/10.1089/lap.2021.0036.

Non-Conservative Management of Chylothorax

18

Hyo Yeong Ahn and Hoseok I

Abstract

Chylothorax is caused by lymphatic leakage, which can develop after thoracic surgery and is associated with cancer. Although prospective randomized trials have not been performed, radiological interventions have been performed in several cases with persistent chylothorax, adjunct to 2 weeks of conservative management. The success rate of such interventions is diverse due to anatomical variations, although the results are promising. However, in cases of treatment failure after cycles of interventions, a team approach may be necessary to determine whether surgical management is warranted.

Keywords

Chylothorax · Management · Intervention Surgery

H. Y. Ahn · H. I (✉)
Department of Thoracic and Cardiovascular Surgery, Pusan National University Hospital, Pusan National University School of Medicine, Biomedical Research Institute, Busan, Republic of Korea
e-mail: ihoseok@pusan.ac.kr

18.1 Introduction

Chylothorax refers to a collection of chyle in the pleural cavity due to leakage from the lymphatic vessels, especially from the thoracic duct. The classification of chylothorax depends on its etiology (traumatic, non-traumatic, or idiopathic). Regardless of the cause, the medical and surgical options to reduce lymph leakage for patients with chylothorax are similar to those for patients with high-flow chylothorax (>25 mL/kg/day) [1–8]. If even repeated interventions are not effective, surgical treatment might be the last option [7, 9, 10]. In the event that surgical management fails, conservative management may be continued until leakage ceases. Unfortunately, the comparison of outcomes between conservative and surgical treatment is limited by the insufficient number of patients with chylothorax for prospective studies to be conducted [7, 8]. In this article, the anatomy of the thoracic duct and the etiology, diagnosis, and treatment of chylothorax are discussed.

18.2 Anatomy

The thoracic duct drains the cisterna chyli, located on the right side of the thoracic vertebrae, which continues on the left from the level of T4 and drains into the left innominate vein (Fig. 18.1). Variations have been observed in more than one-third of the population [2, 9, 11].

K. Kim et al. (eds.), *Techniques in Minimally Invasive Thoracic Surgery*,
https://doi.org/10.1007/978-981-19-2472-9_18

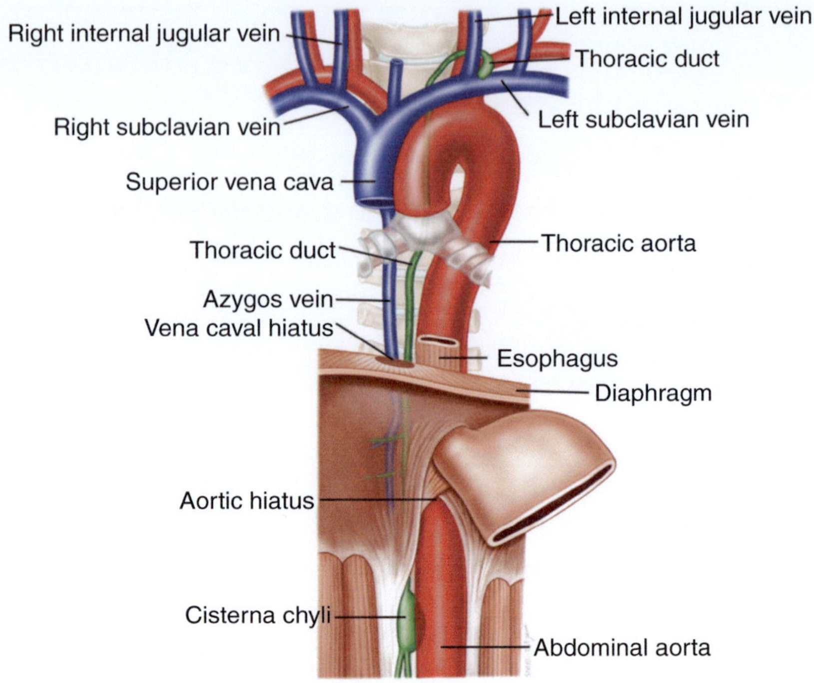

Fig. 18.1 Anatomy of the thoracic duct. From the cisterna chyli, the thoracic duct crosses the diaphragm at the aortic hiatus at the level of the 12th thoracic vertebra, and continues to ascend between the thoracic aorta on the left and the azygos vein on the right. It crosses over to the left side between the fourth and sixth thoracic vertebrae. Finally, it ascends behind the aortic arch and the left subclavian artery

These anatomic variations are the underlying cause of the diversity of intervention success rates [2, 9, 11]. Moreover, there is a high risk of tearing along the course of the lymphatic pathway during esophagectomy and lymph node dissection due to the proximity of the course of the thoracic duct to other structures [1, 12, 13]. Any tear in the thoracic duct can quickly lead to the accumulation of large volumes of lymphatic fluid, since it usually transports around 2–4 L of chyle per day [11].

18.3 Etiology

The etiology of chylothorax can be classified as involving traumatic or non-traumatic injuries to the thoracic duct, although idiopathic chylothorax can also occur [4, 6, 14].

Traumatic Causes (50%)

Direct injury to the thoracic duct, particularly during thoracic surgery (e.g., esophagectomy and lymph node dissection), is the most common cause of traumatic chylothorax. Other traumatic causes include blunt trauma or penetrating injuries [4, 6, 14].

Non-Traumatic Causes (45%)

In cases of non-traumatic chylothorax, direct infiltration or impeded flow caused by compression and accumulation leads to filtration of the lymphatic vessels. Relatively impeded flow can occur if there is increased lymph production, such as in patients with increased central venous pressure or those with liver cirrhosis and portal hypertension. Chylothorax can develop idiopathically in up to 6% of cases [4, 6, 14].

18.4 Diagnosis

The presence of chylomicrons, measuring approximately 0.5–1.0 μm in size, needs to be confirmed in the pleural fluid. Alternatively, chylothorax can be established by triglyceride content >110 mg/dL and a cholesterol concentration <200 mg/dL. A triglyceride concentration of

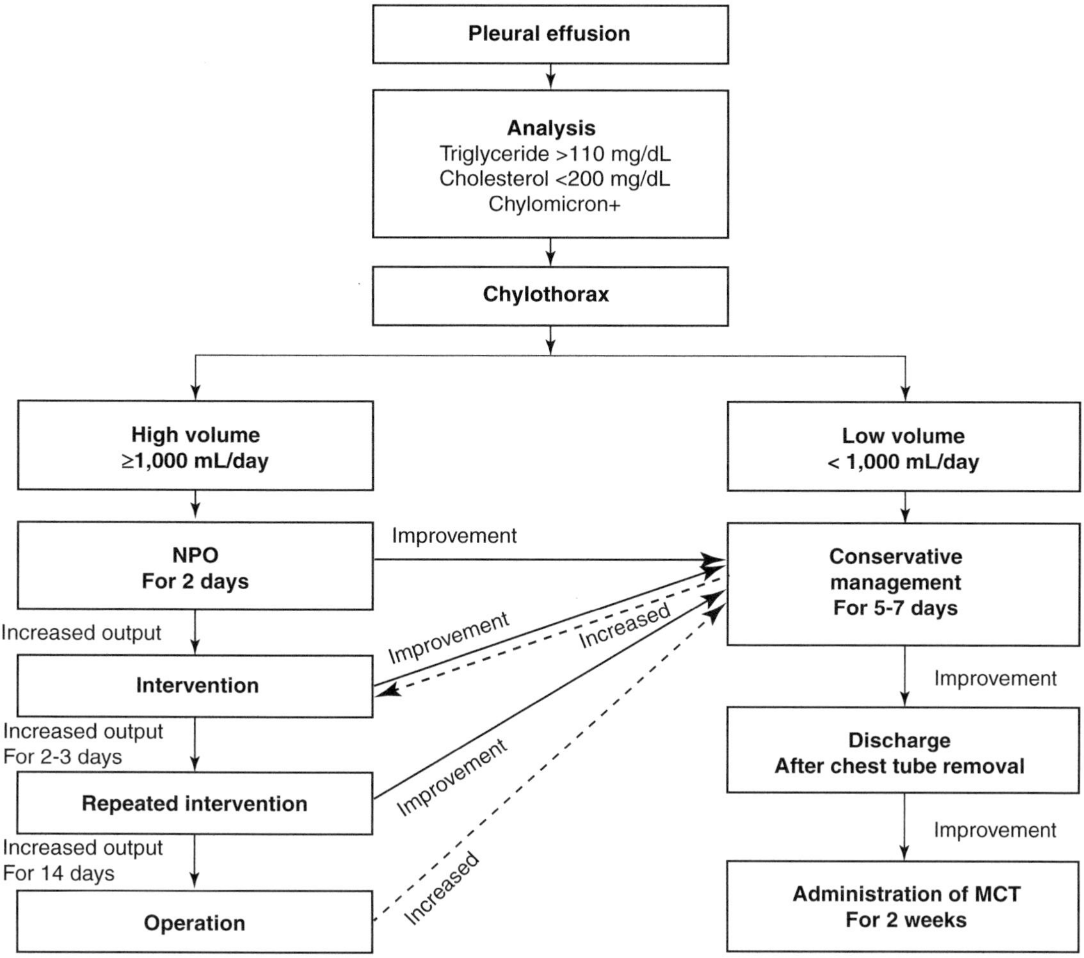

Fig. 18.2 Algorithm of chylothorax management. *MCT* medium-chain triglyceride

<50 mg/dL rules out chylothorax. The differential diagnosis includes pseudochylothorax, which is characterized by low triglyceride content, a cholesterol concentration of >200 mg/dL, and the absence of chylomicrons (Fig. 18.2).

18.5 Treatment

The appropriate treatment method depends on the etiology and amount of chylothorax. Traditionally, conservative treatment is first administered [7, 9, 13–15]. However, in patients with high-volume chylothorax, the timing of appropriate interventions is important. The development of therapeutic methods and an algorithm has ensured a systematic and timely process to deliver treatment (Fig. 18.2). Further randomized trials need to be conducted to establish a consensus on chylothorax management.

Conservative Treatment

Indications

Conservative management is considered the first-line modality for all patients with chylothorax [7, 9, 13–15].

Methods

Nothing by mouth or a diet containing medium-chain triglycerides (MCT) reduces the flow of lymph and may allow spontaneous closure of the leak in the thoracic duct [7, 9]. Adequate fluid and electrolyte replacement with proper nutrition should follow. Additionally, pleural drainage may be done for lung re-expansion and pulmonary function optimization. The administration of octreotide may be considered if drain output persists [16].

Prognosis

The resolution rate after conservative treatment ranges from 16% to more than 75% [7, 9]; however, this figure is lower in patients with high-volume chylothorax (>1000 mL/day). In the event of marked drain output reduction under conservative treatment, a good therapeutic outcome can be achieved after a few weeks of a strict MCT diet.

Interventional Treatment

Indications

Lymphangiography is advisable for almost all patients with persistent chylothorax for the identification of the level of the tear. This applies for both traumatic and non-traumatic chylothorax [4, 6, 11, 16–18].

Methods

Resolution of the thoracic duct leak spontaneously occurs in up to 50% of cases [4, 6, 11]. However, lymphangiography is advisable for the occlusion of chyle fistulas, as has been reported in some cases.

Thoracic Duct Lymphangiography

Thoracic duct lymphangiography, which is performed intranodally via the bilateral inguinal or femoral lymph nodes (Fig. 18.3a–d) [4, 16, 18], requires a 26G needle and a short catheter (Cook, Bloomington, IN, USA) fitted to a luer-lock syringe containing 3–5 mL of lipiodol. Ultrasonography and intermittent fluoroscopy are used to confirm intranodal lymphatic vessel puncture and to guide the subsequent injection of lipiodol at 3 mL/min, respectively. If nodal rupture occurs during the injection, the upper lymph nodes may be directly punctured under fluoroscopic guidance to continue lipiodol administration, which is ceased after the opacification of the lumbar duct or cisterna chyli. The total amount of lipiodol is limited to 20 mL to minimize the risk of pulmonary fat embolism.

Thoracic Duct Embolization

Prior to the procedure, the duct and its adjacent structures (e.g., the aorta) are visualized with cone-beam computed tomography. Thoracic duct embolization is performed by gaining access to the thoracic duct via direct puncture of the lumbar duct or cisterna chyli with a 21G Chiba needle through the transabdominal route [2, 14, 19]. After transabdominal puncture of the cisterna chyli, a 0.018-in. (0.46 mm) Transend guidewire (Boston Scientific Corp., Natick, MA, USA) is used to enter the thoracic duct and is advanced further before the introduction of a 2.0 F or 2.2 F microcatheter (Terumo, Tokyo, Japan), employing an over-the-wire technique (Fig. 18.3e, f). Digital subtraction angiography, aided with a microcatheter, is used to establish the chyle leakage sites, which are then subjected to Concerto microcoil embolization (Medtronic, Jacksonville, FL, USA) proximal to the leakage sites and embolized using a mixture of *N*-butyl cyanoacrylate (NBCA, Histoacryl; B Brown, Melsungen, Germany) and lipiodol (weight ratio 1:1). Coil embolization is done to prevent NBCA migration to the left subclavian vein due to the longer NBCA polymerization time in the lymphatic vessels than in the blood vessels. Lipiodol is injected after establishing needle access to the lymph node. Fluoroscopic images of the cisterna chyli are obtained, and under fluoroscopic guidance, the cisterna chyli is directly punctured using a 21G Chiba needle. A 0.018-in. (0.46 mm) guidewire and microcatheter are used to cannulate the thoracic duct, which is then embolized using Concerto 3EA microcoils and an NBCA/lipiodol mixture (weight ratio 1:1). This procedure has a success rate of over 90% in chylothorax cases [1, 2, 4, 14, 19, 20].

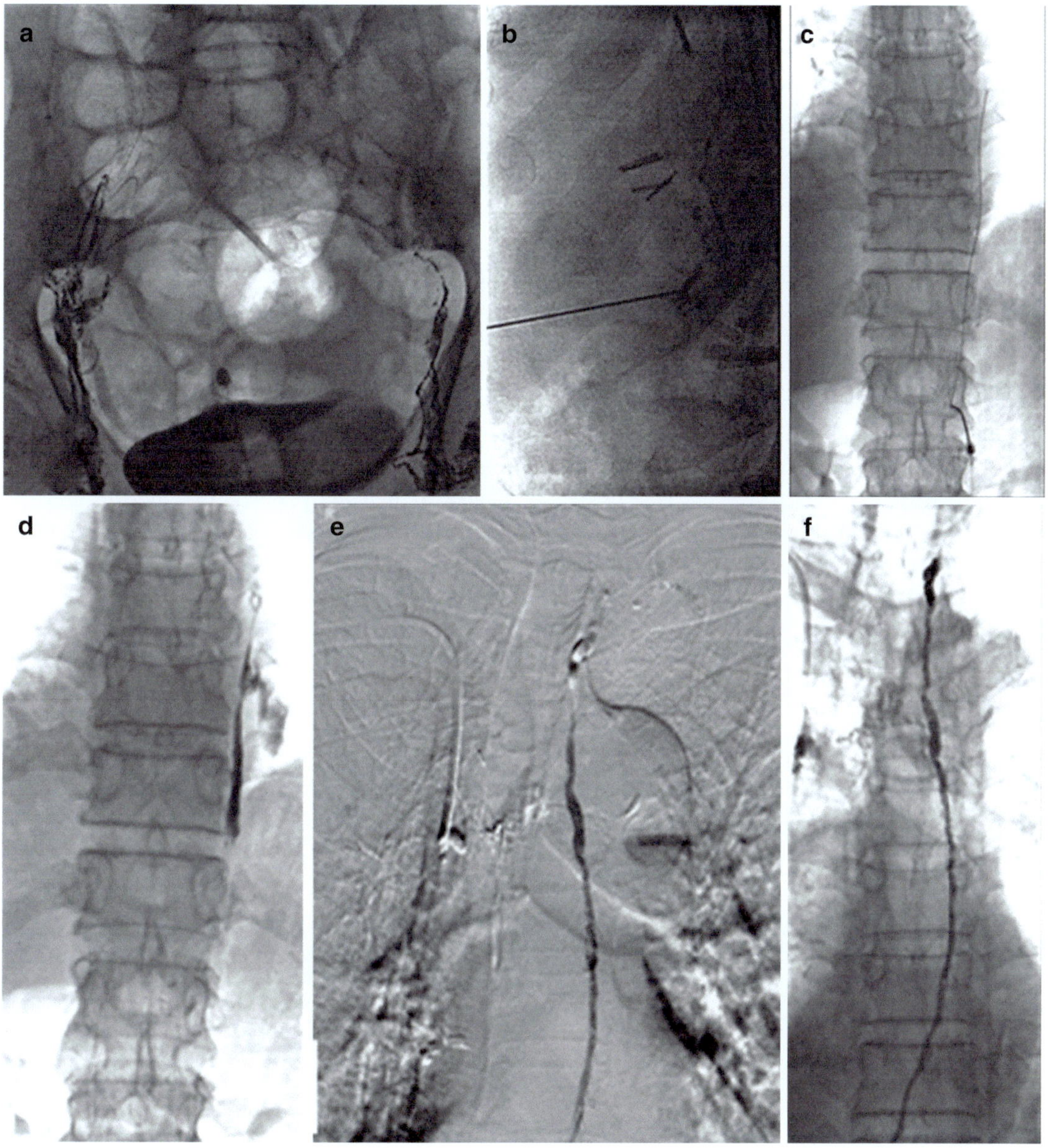

Fig. 18.3 Thoracic duct embolization. (**a**) Intranodal lymphangiography via the bilateral inguinal approach, (**b**) thoracic duct access via direct puncture of the lumbar duct, (**c**) introduction of a microcatheter after insertion of a guidewire, (**d**) digital subtraction angiography to define the chyle leakage site, (**e**) microcoil embolization above the leakage site, and (**f**) embolization using an *N*-butyl cyanoacrylate and lipiodol mixture

Needle Disruption

Needle disruption to reduce lymphatic flow may be performed in cases of small prevertebral lymph vessels, which are anatomic variants in 30% of patients [2].

Transjugular Intrahepatic Portosystemic Stent Shunt

In hepatic chylothorax, transjugular intrahepatic portosystemic shunts may be considered to reduce lymphatic flow [21].

Prognosis

Due to occurrences of non-traumatic chylothorax in patients with underlying diseases, the success rate of interventions is lower than that of traumatic chylothorax [4]. The reported overall success rate in non-traumatic chylothorax management ranges from 27 to 68% [6, 8, 11]. Radiologic intervention might still be considered relatively safe and effective as some studies have reported complication rates of 3% and no critical complications [6, 8, 11].

Surgical Treatment

Indications

Surgery might be the last option if the leak persists for more than 2 weeks, even with conservative treatment or a radiological intervention, or if there is a high-volume chyle leak of more than 1000–1500 mL/day [10, 21–25].

Surgical Methods

Surgical techniques include thoracic duct ligation, mass ligation of the tissue, pleurodesis, and pleuroperitoneal shunting [10, 21–25]. Thoracic duct ligation is performed by ligating or clipping above the right diaphragm, between T8 and T12, regardless of the surgical site (Fig. 18.4). Preoperative administration of olive oil, ice cream, or heavy cream may be done for better identification of the tear site. Alternatively, mass ligation of tissue around the presumed course of the thoracic duct may be considered. As a way to approach the thoracic duct, direct vision might be generally considered; however, in selected cases, video-assisted thoracic surgery could be another option [21, 24, 25]. If the aforementioned operations are not practically feasible, pleurodesis may be performed to induce inflammation and subsequent adhesion between the visceral and parietal pleura. If leakage persists after performing the above-mentioned procedures, insertion of a pleuroperitoneal shunt or external permanent drainage should be considered [10, 21–25].

Prognosis

Generally, surgical interventions have a success rate of approximately 90%, with complications occurring in up to 38.3% of cases [10]. Considerable mortality rates of up to 25% have been reported [10, 25].

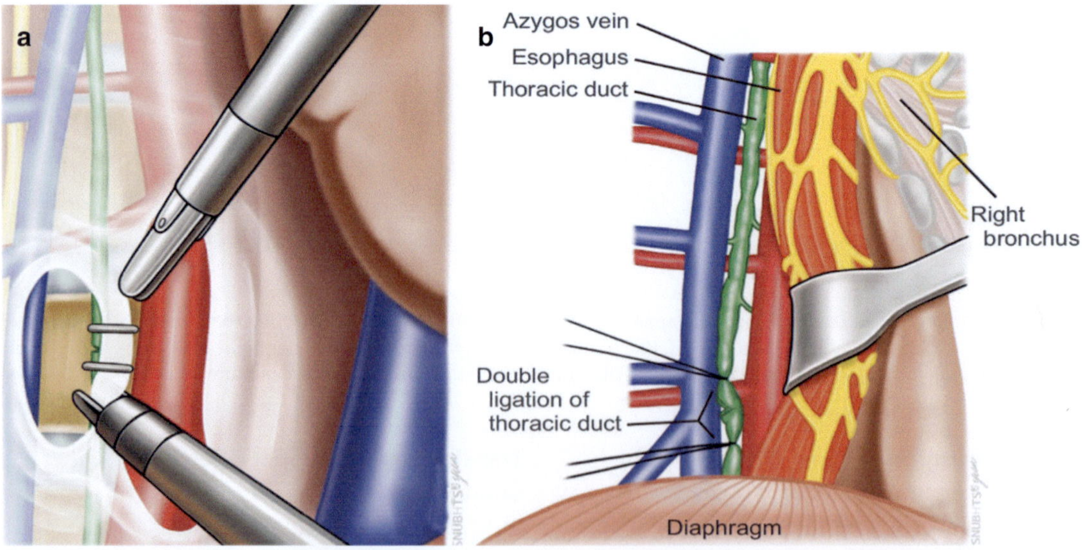

Fig. 18.4 Surgical technique for the treatment of chylothorax. Thoracic duct ligation can be performed by clipping (**a**), or ligation (**b**) above the right diaphragm between T8 and T12

18.6 Conclusion

The development of other interventional methods for chylothorax management is limited by individual competency levels. According to the authors' personal observations in the past 4 years, there is a learning curve for the performance of these procedures at our center. Additionally, anatomic variants of the cisterna chyli or lymphatic vessels have fewer puncture sites to access the thoracic duct for intubation. Nevertheless, lymphangiography remains a promising option for leak resolution [11, 18, 26]. This radiological intervention is considered relatively safe and effective, as shown by its success rate of 52% and complication rate of 3%, without fatal complications [6, 8, 11].

Although radiological interventions have been performed in several cases of persistent chylothorax, whether the outcomes are successful might be affected by the individual radiologist. Therefore, surgeons should be well informed of the anatomy of the thoracic duct, and a team approach may be necessary to determine whether surgical management is warranted in cases of treatment failure after cycles of intervention.

Conflict of Interest No potential conflict of interest relevant to this article was reported.

References

1. Bazancir LA, Jensen RJ, Frevert SC, Ryom P, Achiam MP. Embolization of the thoracic duct in patients with iatrogenic chylothorax. Dis Esophagus. 2021;34(9):doab001. https://doi.org/10.1093/dote/doab001.
2. Binkert CA, Yucel EK, Davison BD, Sugarbaker DJ, Baum RA. Percutaneous treatment of high-output chylothorax with embolization or needle disruption technique. J Vasc Interv Radiol. 2005;16:1257–62.
3. Borcyk K, Kamil A, Hagerty K, Deer M, Tomich P, Anderson Berry AL. Successful management of extremely high-output refractory congenital chylothorax with chemical pleurodesis using 4% povidone–iodine and propranolol: a case report. Clin Case Rep. 2018;6:702–8.
4. Hara H, Mihara M, Yamamoto M. Therapeutic lymphangiography for traumatic chylothorax. J Vasc Surg Venous Lymphat Disord. 2018;6:237–40.
5. Jun H, Hur S. Interventional radiology treatment for postoperative chylothorax. Korean J Thorac Cardiovasc Surg. 2020;53:200–4.
6. Juszczyk K, Waugh R, Sandroussi C. Lymphangiography as therapeutic management of chylothorax. J Med Imaging Radiat Oncol. 2013;57:460–1.
7. Schild HH, Strassburg CP, Welz A, Kalff J. Treatment options in patients with chylothorax. Dtsch Arztebl Int. 2013;110:819–26.
8. Schild HH, Pieper C. Chylothorax: current therapeutic options. Zentralbl Chir. 2019;144:S24–30.
9. Pulle MV, Puri HV, Asaf BB, Bishnoi S, Yadav A, Kumar A. Chylothorax: modalities of management and outcomes: a case series. Lung India. 2021;38:154–60.
10. Tenny BC, Madjarov J, Shipe T. Surgical intervention in a complicated persistent chyle leak. Int J Surg Case Rep. 2018;42:7–9.
11. Matsumoto T, Yamagami T, Kato T, et al. The effectiveness of lymphangiography as a treatment method for various chyle leakages. Br J Radiol. 2009;82:286–90.
12. Tapias LF, Morse CR. A preliminary experience with minimally invasive Ivor Lewis esophagectomy. Dis Esophagus. 2012;25:449–55.
13. Varshney VK, Suman S, Garg PK, Soni SC, Khera PS. Management options for post-esophagectomy chylothorax. Surg Today. 2021;51:678–85.
14. Jeon YJ, Cho JH, Hyun D, et al. Management of chyle leakage after general thoracic surgery: impact of thoracic duct embolization. Thorac Cancer. 2021;12:1382–6.
15. Takuwa T, Yoshida J, Ono S, et al. Low-fat diet management strategy for chylothorax after pulmonary resection and lymph node dissection for primary lung cancer. J Thorac Cardiovasc Surg. 2013;146:571–4.
16. Sharkey AJ, Rao JN. The successful use of octreotide in the treatment of traumatic chylothorax. Tex Heart Inst J. 2012;39:428–30.
17. Nadolski GJ, Itkin M. Lymphangiography and thoracic duct embolization following unsuccessful thoracic duct ligation: imaging findings and outcomes. J Thorac Cardiovasc Surg. 2018;156:838–43.
18. Sommer CM, Pieper CC, Itkin M, et al. Conventional lymphangiography (CL) in the management of postoperative lymphatic leakage (PLL): a systematic review. Rofo. 2020;192:1025–35.
19. Jayasinghe SA, Srinivasa RN, Hage AN, Gemmete JJ, Majdalany BS, Chick JF. Thoracic duct embolization: analysis of practice patterns. Ann Vasc Surg. 2018;52:168–75.
20. Kim PH, Tsauo J, Shin JH. Lymphatic interventions for chylothorax: a systematic review and meta-analysis. J Vasc Interv Radiol. 2018;29:194–202.
21. Lutz P, Strunk H, Schild HH, Sauerbruch T. Transjugular intrahepatic portosystemic shunt in refractory chylothorax due to liver cirrhosis. World J Gastroenterol. 2013;19:1140–2.

22. Arshava EV, Parekh KR. Thoracoscopic thoracic duct ligation: how I teach it. Ann Thorac Surg. 2020;109:1330–4.
23. Liu Z, Du M, Liang Y, Ju S, Li X, Gao Y. Prophylactic ligation of the thoracic duct branch prevents chylothorax after pulmonary resection for right lung cancer. Surg Today. 2020;50:881–8.
24. Yamagata Y, Saito K, Hirano K, Oya M. Laparoscopic transhiatal thoracic duct ligation for chylothorax after esophagectomy. Thorac Cardiovasc Surg. 2019;67:606–9.
25. Yang RF, Liu TT, Wang P, et al. Ligation of thoracic duct during thoracoscopic esophagectomy can lead to decrease of T lymphocyte. J Cancer Res Ther. 2018;14:1535–9.
26. Yamagami T, Masunami T, Kato T, et al. Spontaneous healing of chyle leakage after lymphangiography. Br J Radiol. 2005;78:854–7.

19 Non-Intubated Video-Assisted Thoracic Surgery

Kyung Soo Kim and Won Jung Hwang

Abstract

Non-intubated VATS (NIVATS) is a surgical method that is performed under the patient's spontaneous respiration without tracheal intubation. NIVATS reduces adverse effects such as ventilator-induced lung injury from mechanical ventilation and induces a faster recovery. In order to safely perform NIVATS, appropriate patient selection, assessment, and a multidisciplinary team approach are required.

19.1 Introduction

Video-assisted thoracoscopic surgery (VATS) has been evolved by technical innovations and instrumental developments. Thus, most of thoracic surgeries were initiated under thoracoscopic settings, even requiring complex procedures. Moreover, reduced port surgery has been demonstrating efficacy with acceptable outcomes, compared to multi-port VATS or thoracotomy. In accordance with minimally invasive trends, non-intubated thoracoscopic surgeries has also been increasingly employed with VATS experiences. Non-intubated VATS (NIVATS) which comprises maintenance of spontaneous respiration without tracheal intubation for one-lung ventilation has revealed feasibility and benefits of less invasiveness [1, 2]. Expected rewards are explained by removal of adverse effects from mechanical ventilation, which includes intubation injury or lung damages. Moreover, adequate loco-regional block has been offered grants, avoiding potential harmful effects of neuromuscular blockade, that rapid recovery is observed with reduced usage of sedative and analgesics [3]. Shortened induction and recovery time enables reduced total operation time that urinary catheter and central venous catheter can be omitted. Finally, fast postoperative recovery facilitates patients discharge earlier with better quality of life, compared to intubated VATS [4]. Routine drainage tubes also can be deleted for entirely tubeless VATS settings to decrease postoperative pain [5]. To initiate and set up the NIVATS protocol, proper indications and experienced team approach are mandatory. With flexibility, NIVATS should be changed to intubation settings whenever surgeons or anesthesiologist demands to keep on safety operations. Understanding basic steps and strategy is essential to recognize NIVATS, as a promising alternative for conventional intubated VATS.

K. S. Kim (✉)
Department of Thoracic and Cardiovascular Surgery, Seoul St. Mary's Hospital, The Catholic University of Korea, Seoul, Republic of Korea
e-mail: cskks@catholic.ac.kr

W. J. Hwang
Department of Anesthesia and Pain Medicine, Seoul St. Mary's Hospital, The Catholic University of Korea, Seoul, Republic of Korea

K. Kim et al. (eds.), *Techniques in Minimally Invasive Thoracic Surgery*,
https://doi.org/10.1007/978-981-19-2472-9_19

19.2 Pathophysiological Changes During NIVATS

In the spontaneous respiration cycle, the lung expands due to the negative pressure in the closed chest cavity during inspiration. During NIVATS, the concept is to allow the creation of a "surgical pneumothorax" as the surgeon opens the chest [6]. Once thorax cavity is opened with surgical incision, the negative pressure is lost. Therefore, the lung cannot expand during spontaneous breathing, resulting in lung collapse. Further lung collapse is promoted by the external atmospheric pressure. This can provide excellent lung isolation without the need for positive pressure ventilation on the dependent lung. However, respiratory and hemodynamic derangement may also occur due to two major physiologic changes after surgical pneumothorax. First, both lungs are not completely separated during NIVATS. Therefore, part of the air inside the non-operated lung enters into the surgical lung during expiration, causing CO_2 rebreathing. Converse flow occurs during inspiration, and it contributes to lung collapse of surgical site. This is called "paradoxical respiration," which commonly makes hypoxia and hypercapnia during NIVATS [7]. Second, mediastinal structure swings according to the respiratory cycle and moves downward by gravity, which may cause hemodynamic instability and decrease the dependent lung to offer efficient tidal volume.

Oxygenation in NIVATS is well maintained in properly selected patients because *V*/*Q* mismatch is reduced with hypoxic pulmonary vasoconstriction, the lateral position, and relatively preserved FRC and the diaphragm function. Hypoxia may occur in patients with impaired pulmonary function, but most of them improve with increasing oxygen flow. Hypercapnia is a more common problem because CO_2 rebreathing occurs during paradoxical respiration and respiratory depression is caused by the use of sedative and opioid. However, the concept of permissive hypercapnia is applied to one-lung ventilation, and it is considered safe to reach 70 mmHg $PaCO_2$. Breathing increases with postoperative awakening, and CO_2 concentration is restored to normal range.

19.3 Challenging Indications

Patients having poor pulmonary functions have been selectively decided for VATS under spontaneous ventilation to avoid ventilator-induced lung injury [8, 9]. With evolving NIVATS procedures, variety of thoracic procedures have been reported under non-intubated settings with modifying VATS approaches, simple procedures for pleural disease, hyperhidrosis, pneumothorax, pulmonary nodules, and mediastinal tumors [10–12]. Nowadays, VATS has become the standard surgical modality for early lung cancers. Oncologic advantages after lung cancer surgery under NIVATS have also been endorsed [13, 14]. Moreover, technically demanding cases of tracheal resection and sleeve lobectomy were also reported [15, 16]. However, any unstable conditions of patient intolerance may happen by surgical or anesthetic events with inexperience. Above all, surgical team should recognize the physiology of non-intubated anesthesia. Proper selection is emphasized of patients with ECOG performance status less than 1, anesthesiologist standard (ASA) grade less than II, and low BMI less than 25 kg/m^2 [17]. Patients with expected difficult airway are absolutely contraindicated because of the high incidence of hypoxemia and the possibility of intraoperative intubation failure. Previous history of pleural infection or thoracic surgery having possibility of dense adhesions might be relatively contraindicated because it is difficult to perform intraoperative intercostal block. Patients with significant cardiopulmonary dysfunction or neurologic deficit also will be excluded due to possibility of hemodynamic collapse with severe hypercarbia. In planning difficult thoracic procedures, cooperation with anesthesiologist under cautious monitoring is more essential, and underlying morbidities should be discussed with consultants preoperatively. With experienced team settings, tubeless, uniportal VATS has been introduced in lung cancer surgery [18, 19].

19.4 Anesthetic Perspectives

General evaluation studies are compatible with traditional VATS under one-lung ventilation. Pulmonary function test, echocardiography, and arterial blood gas analysis on resting status are listed for checkup. Especially, anticipated difficult airway, obesity, and expected extensive pleural adhesions due to history of severe infectious disease or prior thoracic surgery are thoroughly assessed for proper patient selection [20].

In addition to standard monitoring (included non-invasive blood pressure, SpO_2, and ECG), end-tidal CO_2 ($ETCO_2$) and invasive arterial blood pressure monitoring are in place to monitor real-time respiration and hemodynamic changes. Bispectral index (BIS) is highly recommended for evaluation of sedation level and advanced judgement of anesthetic depth, aiming for BIS over 40–60. The level of sedation should be selected according to the patient's condition and type of surgery. Simple procedures (i.e., lung biopsy or pleurodesis) in patients with poor pulmonary function may be performed under full awake state with neuraxial block. Moderate or deep sedation is necessary for the patient's comfort, especially in the prolonged procedure like lobectomy, which makes it intolerable to maintain same position for several hours. Omitting endotracheal intubation, total intravenous anesthesia is introduced for sedation without use of muscle relaxant under loco-regional block with modifications [21]. Continuous infusion of propofol with/without remifentanil using target-controlled infusion (TCI) would mostly create a balanced status with sufficient sedation and ventilatory/hemodynamic stability. Dexmedetomidine can be used as a good alternative or adjuvant for continuous infusion. In the case of sedation, we should monitor the level of consciousness and the pattern of breathing with BIS and $ETCO_2$, respectively. The goal of ventilation management is to maintain a smooth and non-effort respiratory pattern with respiratory rate over 12–20 times/minute for providing a satisfactory surgical field. Meticulous modification of infusion rate or adjuvant administration of fentanyl, midazolam, and ketamine is required to maintain proper range of BIS and breathing [22]. Various loco-regional anesthesia is used for analgesia covering chest cage and parietal pleura. Thoracic epidural block, paravertebral nerve block, and thoracoscopic intercostal nerve blocks are useful in intrapleural analgesia. Vagus nerve block can minimize irritating sensation from visceral pleura and prevent cough reflex during surgical manipulation.

Oxygenation could be facilitated with O_2 supplement by nasal cannula or by facial mask (Fig. 19.1). In patients with poor pulmonary function requiring deep sedation, supraglottic

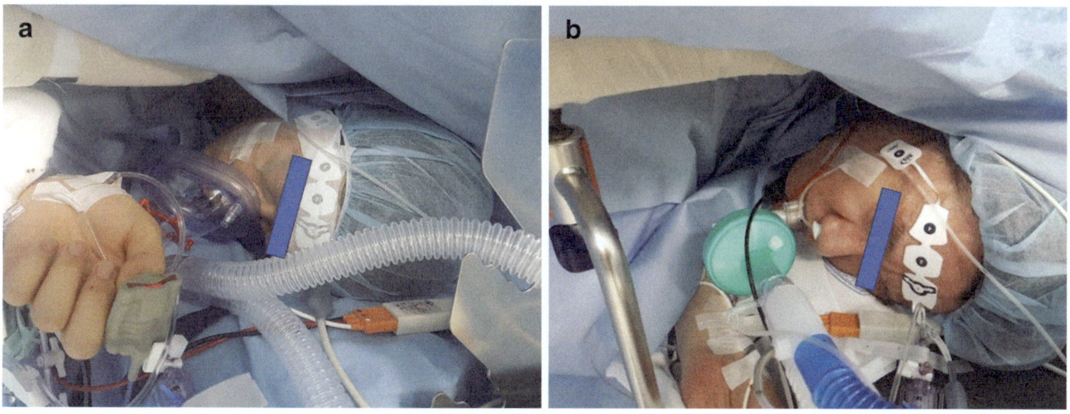

Fig. 19.1 Oxygenation with facial mask (**a**) or laryngeal mask (**b**)

device such as laryngeal mask airway (LMA) can be useful. If SpO_2 drops to below 90% or $PaCO_2$ increases over 60 mmHg, infusion rates of anesthetic agents are modified, and temporary mechanical or assisted ventilation is applied. When unstable condition is not controlled, conversion to endotracheal intubation should be assessed. Position change for semi-lateral decubitus or supine position is required to assess adequate airway management. Single lumen tube with bronchial blocker or double-lumen endotracheal tube can be replaced under guidance of video-laryngoscope and/or fiberoptic bronchoscope. Intubation related oral, tracheal, and tooth injuries might be occurring that should be announced preoperatively.

19.5 Surgical Perspectives

Thoracoscopic procedures are usually equivocal to conventional intubated VATS according to surgeon's preferences. Under lateral decubitus positioning with sterilization, transparent draping between surgical field and anesthesiologist offers benefits for cooperative monitoring. Ultrasound-guided paravertebral (or epidural) block is made preoperatively. Preemptive anesthetic local injection is given in placing thoracoscopic working wound with ports placement, avoiding compression of the thoracic cage (Fig. 19.2a). Entering the thoracic cavity, surgical pneumothorax was identified, and intercostal (T2–T9 levels) nerve block is introduced under lung collapse if preoperative neuraxial block is not performed (Fig. 19.2b). Vagal nerve block is applied over the mediastinal pleural region around the trachea above the azygos vein for right sided, and below the aortic arch for the left sided to prevent cough reflex (Fig. 19.2c, d). Local anesthetic spray on pharyngeal cavity, inhaled lidocaine or satellite ganglion block also may be applied. Irritations to intrathoracic structures increase the risk of coughing reflex causing mediastinal or diaphragm bulging. Thus, gentle manipulation during pulling or retraction of the lung, bronchial tree, and hilum is essential for surgeons and assistants. During procedures, additional vagal block or regional anesthesia over pleural surfaces might be required if the surgical field is not suitable due to persistent coughing or excessive lung movement from deep breathing. After completing the thoracic procedure, the anesthesiologist performs manual positive pressure ventilation with mask fitting to achieve both lung inflation, allowing an air leak test or two lung ventilation. Air vent is more attained using temporary negative pressure maneuver through the drainage tube or catheter for lung recruitment. During sealing the VATS wounds, the chest tube can be placed with continuous negative pressure or can be removed after tightening of last suturing immediately for chest tubeless VATS. Postoperatively, NIVATS preserves physiologic cardiopulmonary function and neurologic status that stable fast recovery can be realized with less common nausea or vomiting symptoms. Atelectasis or effusion may occur due to mucus plugging in bronchial airways and incomplete lung expansion. Encouraging deep breathing and cough is mandatory as alike as conventional VATS for respiratory toileting.

In cases requiring irritating manipulation causing refractory cough reflex, decision should be made whether to continue NIVATS with sedation control, or to convert into endotracheal intubation. If abrupt inflation of the lung or sudden mediastinal bulging continues, withdrawals of thoracoscopic instruments from the surgical fields be promptly executed to avoid intrathoracic organ or intercostal injury. Minor bleedings or injuries can be managed with suturing, coagulation or sealing materials as preferred thoracoscopic techniques. Conversion is required for treating invasive tumor characteristics or severe pleura and hilar adhesions with anthracosis. Smooth conversion is properly carried out under hemostatic compression, and situations of major bleeding may need emergent thoracotomy. This also have to be settled in respiratory distress with intractable arrhythmia despite of modifying ventilation setting [23]. Continuing NIVATS should be reassessed for time-consuming unsafe procedures, not to make catastrophic situa-

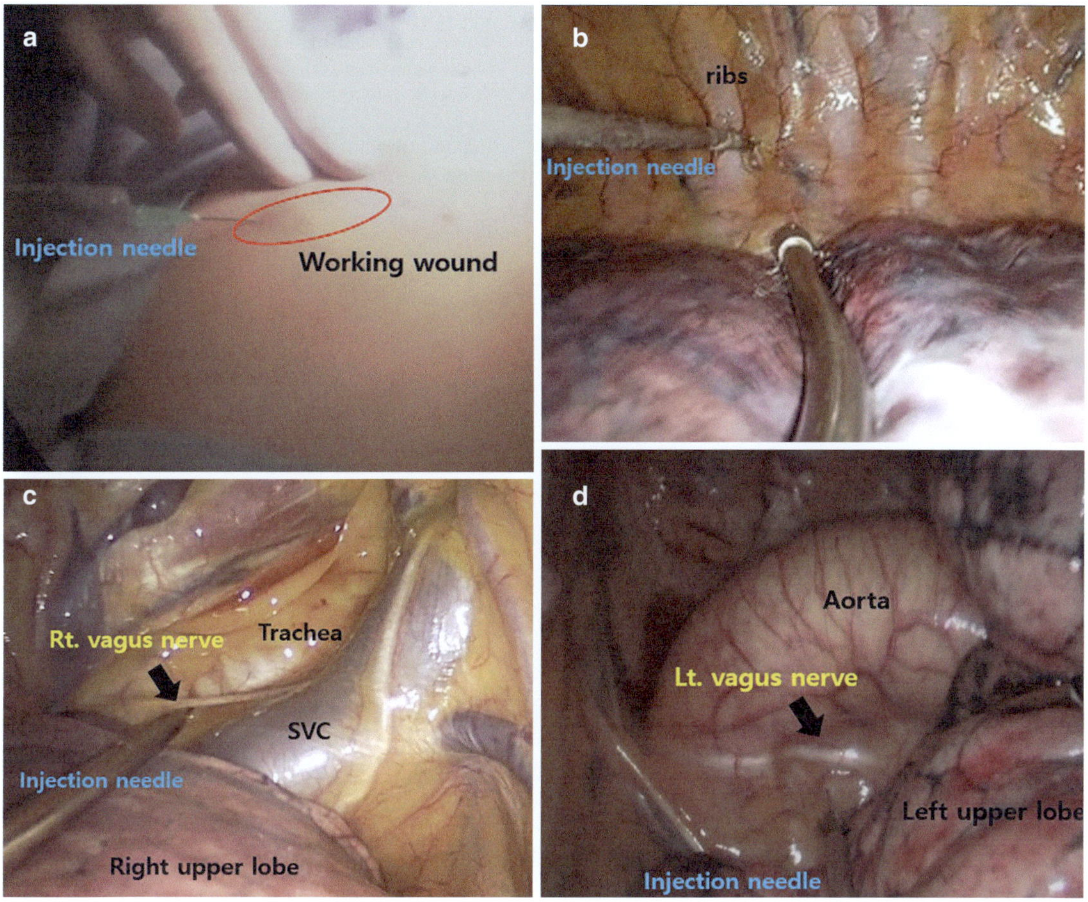

Fig. 19.2 Preemptive anesthetic local injection (**a**) and intercostal nerve block (**b**) and right sided (**c**) and left sided (**d**) vagal block during uniportal approach

tions of major vessel bleeding and to complete complex procedures [24]. Developing NIVATS techniques with proper patient selections have been demonstrated as effectively applicable substitutes or modification to conventional VATS that promisingly suggested [25]. Focus in performing NIVATS is continuous interactions with the anesthesiologist, as dedicated team surgery. Educational simulation program under protocol is essential to avoid uneventful situations, even for simple procedures by proper selection criteria. Resonable consensus protocol is still expected to reveal the exact role of NIVATS on morbidities and oncological issues with extended indications for thoracic diseases.

19.6 Conclusion

NIVATS has revealed effectiveness as alternative, less invasive procedure in treating variable thoracic diseases. Reduced postoperative complication and faster recovery have proved its feasibility and efficacy compared to conventional intubated VATS. To set up and conduct NIVATS safely, dedicated team approach and patient-specific assessment are important in both thoracic surgery and anesthetic fields.

Conflict of Interest No potential conflict of interest relevant to this article was reported.

References

1. Mineo TC, Tacconi F. From "awake" to "monitored anesthesia care" thoracic surgery: a 15 year evolution. Thorac Cancer. 2014;5(1):1–13.
2. Pompeo E, Mineo D, Rogliani P, Sabato AF, Mineo TC. Feasibility and results of awake thoracoscopic resection of solitary pulmonary nodules. Ann Thorac Surg. 2004;78(5):1761–8.
3. Lan L, Cen Y, Zhang C, Qiu Y, Ouyang B. A propensity score-matched analysis for non-intubated thoracic surgery. Med Sci Monit. 2018;24:8081–7.
4. Zhang XX, Song CT, Gao Z, Zhou B, Wang HB, Gong Q, et al. A comparison of non-intubated video-assisted thoracic surgery with spontaneous ventilation and intubated video-assisted thoracic surgery: a meta-analysis based on 14 randomized controlled trials. J Thorac Dis. 2021;13(3):1624–40.
5. Cui F, Liu J, Li S, Yin W, Xin X, Shao W, et al. Tubeless video-assisted thoracoscopic surgery (VATS) under non-intubated, intravenous anesthesia with spontaneous ventilation and no placement of chest tube post-operatively. J Thorac Dis. 2016;8(8):2226–32.
6. David P, Pompeo E, Fabbi E, Dauri M. Surgical pneumothorax under spontaneous ventilation-effect on oxygenation and ventilation. Ann Transl Med. 2015;3(8):106.
7. Liu YJ, Hung MH, Hsu HH, Chen JS, Cheng YJ. Effects on respiration of nonintubated anesthesia in thoracoscopic surgery under spontaneous ventilation. Ann Transl Med. 2015;3(8):107.
8. Peng G, Liu M, Luo Q, Chen H, Yin W, Wang W, et al. Spontaneous ventilation anesthesia combined with uniportal and tubeless thoracoscopic lung biopsy in selected patients with interstitial lung diseases. J Thorac Dis. 2017;9(11):4494–501.
9. Pompeo E, Rogliani P, Atinkaya C, Guerrera F, Ruffini E, Iniguez-Garcia MA, et al. Nonintubated surgical biopsy of undetermined interstitial lung disease: a multicentre outcome analysis. Interact Cardiovasc Thorac Surg. 2019;28(5):744–50.
10. Liang H, Liu J, Wu S, Zhang Y, Liu H, Yang H, et al. Nonintubated spontaneous ventilation offers better short-term outcome for mediastinal tumor surgery. Ann Thorac Surg. 2019;108(4):1045–51.
11. Zhang K, Chen HG, Wu WB, Li XJ, Wu YH, Xu JN, et al. Non-intubated video-assisted thoracoscopic surgery vs. intubated video-assisted thoracoscopic surgery for thoracic disease: a systematic review and meta-analysis of 1684 cases. J Thorac Dis. 2019;11(8):3556–68.
12. Elkhouly A, Pompeo E. Nonintubated subxiphoid bilateral redo lung volume reduction surgery. Ann Thorac Surg. 2018;106(5):e277–e9.
13. Liu J, Cui F, Pompeo E, Gonzalez-Rivas D, Chen H, Yin W, et al. The impact of non-intubated versus intubated anaesthesia on early outcomes of video-assisted thoracoscopic anatomical resection in non-small-cell lung cancer: a propensity score matching analysis. Eur J Cardiothorac Surg. 2016;50(5):920–5.
14. Furák J, Paróczai D, Burián K, Szabó Z, Zombori T. Oncological advantage of nonintubated thoracic surgery: better compliance of adjuvant treatment after lung lobectomy. Thorac Cancer. 2020;11(11):3309–16.
15. Peng G, Cui F, Ang KL, Zhang X, Yin W, Shao W, et al. Non-intubated combined with video-assisted thoracoscopic in carinal reconstruction. J Thorac Dis. 2016;8(3):586–93.
16. Jiang L, Liu J, Gonzalez-Rivas D, Shargall Y, Kolb M, Shao W, et al. Thoracoscopic surgery for tracheal and carinal resection and reconstruction under spontaneous ventilation. J Thorac Cardiovasc Surg. 2018;155(6):2746–54.
17. Li S, Jiang L, Ang KL, Chen H, Dong Q, Yang H, et al. New tubeless video-assisted thoracoscopic surgery for small pulmonary nodules. Eur J Cardiothorac Surg. 2017;51(4):689–93.
18. Gonzalez-Rivas D, Yang Y, Guido W, Jiang G. Non-intubated (tubeless) uniportal video-assisted thoracoscopic lobectomy. Ann Cardiothorac Surg. 2016;5(2):151–3.
19. Liu CY, Hsu PK, Chien HC, Hsieh CC, Ting CK, Tsou MY. Tubeless single-port thoracoscopic sublobar resection: indication and safety. J Thorac Dis. 2018;10(6):3729–37.
20. He J, Liu J, Zhu C, Dai T, Cai K, Zhang Z, et al. Expert consensus on tubeless video-assisted thoracoscopic surgery (Guangzhou). J Thorac Dis. 2019;11(10):4101–8.
21. Mogahed MM, Elkahwagy MS. Paravertebral block versus intercostal nerve block in non-intubated uniportal video-assisted thoracoscopic surgery: a randomised controlled trial. Heart Lung Circ. 2020;29(5):800–7.
22. Irons JF, Martinez G. Anaesthetic considerations for non-intubated thoracic surgery. J Visc Surg. 2016;2:61.
23. Lirio F, Galvez C, Bolufer S, Corcoles JM, Gonzalez-Rivas D. Tubeless major pulmonary resections. J Thorac Dis. 2018;10(Suppl 22):S2664–S70.
24. Hung WT, Hung MH, Wang ML, Cheng YJ, Hsu HH, Chen JS. Nonintubated thoracoscopic surgery for lung tumor: seven years' experience with 1025 patients. Ann Thorac Surg. 2019;107(6):1607–12.
25. Gonzalez-Rivas D, Bonome C, Fieira E, Aymerich H, Fernandez R, Delgado M, et al. Non-intubated video-assisted thoracoscopic lung resections: the future of thoracic surgery? Eur J Cardiothorac Surg. 2016;49(3):721–31.

MIX
Papier aus verantwortungsvollen Quellen
Paper from responsible sources
FSC® C105338

If you have any concerns about our products,
you can contact us on
ProductSafety@springernature.com

In case Publisher is established outside the EU,
the EU authorized representative is:
Springer Nature Customer Service Center GmbH
Europaplatz 3, 69115 Heidelberg, Germany

Printed by Libri Plureos GmbH
in Hamburg, Germany